The Role of the Mental Health Nurse

Edited by

Sheila Forster
Senior Lecturer in Mental Health
Canterbury Christ Church University College

First published in 2001 by:
Nelson Thornes Ltd
Delta Place
27 Bath Road
CHELTENHAM
Glos GL53 7TH
United Kingdom

Set in 10/12pt Classical Garamond

01 02 03 04 05 / 10 9 8 7 6 5 4 3 2 1

A catalogue record for this book is available from the British Library

ISBN 0 7487 3893 2

Typeset by Acorn Bookwork, Salisbury, Wiltshire
Printed and bound in Great Britain by T.J. International Ltd, Padstow, Cornwall

CONTENTS

LIST OF CONTRIBUTORS

Mohammed Abuel Ealeh MSc(Nursing), BEd, DipN, DipNEd, RNT, RMN, RGN, MHSM
Principal Lecturer and Head of Mental Health Division, Anglia Polytechnic University, Chelmsford, Essex

Richard Barrett BA(Hons), MA, RMN, RNT, DipN
Senior Lecturer, Anglia Polytechnic University, Chelmsford, Essex

Stuart Donald
Community Psychiatric Nurse, East Kent Community Trust, Deal, Kent

Sheila Forster CertEd, BEd, MEd, RMN, DipCPN, RNT, DipCouns
Senior Lecturer in Mental Health, Canterbury Christ Church University College, Canterbury, Kent

Rob Lancaster RMN, BA, MA, CPN Cert
Locality Manager, East Kent Community Trust, Dover, Kent

Tony Leiba PhD, MPhil, MSc, BA, DipN, RMN, RNT
Lecturer, City University, London

Norman MacDonald MA, RMN, DipCPN, PGDipEd
Senior Lecturer in Mental Health, Harold Wood Hospital, Harold Wood, Essex

Doug MacInnes RMN, BSc(Hons), PhD
Senior Lecturer in Mental Health, Canterbury Christ Church University College, Canterbury, Kent

Matthew Morrissey BSc, MSc, RMN, DipEd, PGCE, RNT
Senior Lecturer in Mental Health, Canterbury Christ Church University College, Canterbury, Kent

Andrew Thomas RMN, RGN, RCNT, DipNEd, RNT, BEd(Hons), MSc(Nursing)
Senior Lecturer in Mental Health, Canterbury Christ Church University College, Canterbury, Kent

Mark Wilbourn RMN, BSc(Hons)
Senior Lecturer in Mental Health, Canterbury Christ Church University College, Canterbury, Kent

FOREWORD

Whereas other professionals will see atypical, socially unacceptable behaviours as symptomatic of disease, psychiatric nurses occupy a role in which they recognize such behaviours as problem-solving actions, emblematic of difficulties arising within interpersonal relationships. The impetus for this book was from practitioners who wanted to express their understanding of the personal meaning, context and role of psychiatric care, to offer informed descriptions of the roles of the mental health nurse for entry-level students and practitioners.

The Role of the Mental Health Nurse is a fitting tribute to a profession which finds growing consensus in the interpersonal skills put forward by Hilda Peplau, who died in 1999 following a momentous contribution to psychiatric nursing. The time could not be better for a book which sets about establishing a 'how-to' stall and also provides a fitting commemoration of initiatives in new directions for practice and professional development (DoH 1999a,b, Peach 1999, Peplau 1999). Many books set out to be *the* text on psych-conditions for nurses, on history, on theory and so on; that somehow practice will follow theory. The tacit ambition of this book is to describe how clinical and teaching practice is theory; theory in the making, 'making it' from the bottom up in a context of practical and theoretical guides, as far as psychiatric and mental health nursing is concerned.

Professor Bill Lemmer
Canterbury Christ Church University College

REFERENCES

DoH (1999a) *Making a Difference*. Department of Health, London.
DoH (1999b) *A National Service Framework for Mental Health*. Department of Health, London.
Peach, L. (1999) *Fitness for Practice*. United Kingdom Central Council, London.
Peplau, H.E. (1999) Psychotherapeutic strategies. *Perspectives in Psychiatric Care* 35(3).

PREFACE

This book does not claim to be an exhaustive inventory of all the roles of the mental health nurse since we recognize that, due to individual styles, skills and preferences, nurses soon after qualifying may choose to extend their range of clinical experiences into new areas. However, we have attempted to present the underlying themes which we believe are at the heart of mental health nursing.

Each chapter presents a different facet of this nursing but it must be stressed that the thread that runs right through this book is that of questioning how the large body of theory pertaining to mental health nursing can be applied to care on an individual basis, which is why each chapter moves from theory to its application in practice. For example, what is the point in being able to quote verbatim from theories of supervision unless student nurses and their mentors can then reach agreement on how they want to use, and gain benefit from, the clinical supervision time that they share? Similarly, what is the use of keeping a reflective journal unless learning and new insights into patient care arise as a result?

We hope that the reader will be able to use any or all of the chapters to identify their own best practice, to question their developing skills and to avoid stereotyped ideas and practices which can act to the detriment of the patient.

Sheila Forster

1 AN INTRODUCTION TO THE HISTORY OF MENTAL HEALTH NURSING

Tony Leiba

OBJECTIVES

After reading this chapter, you should be able to:

- map the development of mental health nursing and the changes to the role of the mental health nurse from the Middle Ages to the present day
- understand the changes in the way the mentally ill are perceived and the resulting alterations in the nature of the care they are given
- identify key legislation affecting the role of the mental health nurse and the provision of care to the mentally ill.

This chapter will look at the development of mental health nursing and the changes inherent in the role of those who care for the mentally ill. The reader will be able to trace the growth over several centuries of the underlying idea that those being cared for were not 'mad sinners' but rather people who needed care and understanding.

THE MIDDLE AGES

The men and women who cared for the 'mad', the 'lunatic', the 'insane' or the 'mentally ill' have had a long history and a variety of names. In the Middle Ages care was provided by a worker called 'master', a priest who appointed people to administer to the needs of the 'insane' in special institutions. These special institutions, known as 'hospitals', were ecclesiastical and not medical institutions. They were for care rather than cure, for the relief of the body and the refreshment of the soul by religious observances. The earliest charitable 'hospitals' in England were the 'houses of hospitality'. In about the year 1148 St Bartholomew's in Smithfields was the place where sick pilgrims found relief. There were also other institutions such as hostels, monastic houses and lazar houses where the 'insane' were received. The founders and benefactors of these institutions were often royalty, benevolent bishops, merchants and leading townsfolk.

The first mention of a care worker was the master, who was required to visit, to console and to confer upon patients the sacraments of the church. In the leper houses the master himself might be a leper who managed the affairs of the institution and supervised the workers who were called leper guardians and leper wardens. In some houses which were dependent upon a monastery, a monk was usually selected to superintend the house. The monks also collected alms to help with the financial upkeep of the houses. These monks were also called basketmen because they walked with baskets to collect alms. Employed within those houses were men and women who worked as domestics, laundry women, cooks, servants and carers for the bedridden, called brethren and sisters. In the almshouses, the master was also known as warden custos, keeper or rector. Usually he was a priest but occasionally a layman.

All appointments were usually in the hands of the patrons and staff and inmates were admitted by a religious ceremony. Internal authority was vested in the master or warden whose power was sometimes absolute. External super-vision was dependent upon the patron or his agent, who was supposed to inspect the premises and the accounts annually. Punishment inflicted on inmates and staff consisted of: flogging, fasting, fines, stocks, suspensions and expulsions. Custody for those who proved too violent or unmanageable in the community was provided by the local gaol. The insane were admitted to the same houses and hospitals as people who were diseased in body; they were not even accom-modated in different wards.

It is not known when the separation occurred but the first hospital to become famous in England as a refuge for the insane was Bethlem Hospital at Bishopsgate in London. The house of Bethlem was originally founded as a convent by Simon Fitzmary in 1247. Apart from the insane, the poor, vagrants and beggars who roamed the streets were thought to be in need of control and surveillance. Bridewells or houses of correction were developed to contain them and one in London was linked administratively to the Bethlem. In the bridewells and Bethlem at the time were workers called beadles who were involved in the safe custody of inmates. At this stage insanity was not linked to medicine but rather to religion, correction and discipline.

From a legal point of view a distinction was drawn at an early period between lunatics and idiots. The legislative provision for the protection of their estates was made in the statute *de Praerogative Regis* of 1312. Edwards (1975) and Jones (1955) argued that this was probably the first mental health legislation. This statute recognized the distinction between a lunatic or person of unsound mind and an idiot or natural fool. Its main preoccupation, however, was with the estates of lunatics and idiots rather than with the care and maintenance of the persons themselves. In the case of lunatics, the profits from their lands and tenements were to provide for their necessities and be kept so that they might be restored to them on recovery or given to their heirs on death. In the case of idiots, the profits from their lands were to provide for their necessities, and after their death their lands would go to their rightful heirs. Such persons were kept in custody mainly in houses owned by private individuals and were subjected to little supervision.

THE 16TH AND 17TH CENTURIES

Between the Middle Ages and the Industrial Revolution, the insane were either wanderers from place to place in search of alms or inmates in a house of correction, bridewell, hospital or hostel. Men were divided from women in these institutions and they were overcrowded and poorly ventilated. The workers with the insane, basketmen and keepers, were governed by rule books which listed the tasks which the staff were expected to perform and how inmates ought to be treated. The rules outlined what the governors expected of the staff, the framework for the organization of activities with the inmates and the boundaries for day-to-day activities. They covered routine and order, surveillance and discipline and showed where power lay and the sanctions and disciplinary actions which might be taken.

In 1537 the Order of the Hospitals of Henry VIII and Edward VI was published for the royal hospitals of London, namely St Bartholomew's, Christ's, Bethlem, Bridewell and St Thomas's. The Order detailed the charge given to each of the officers of these hospitals, including the matrons, basketmen, keepers, gallery maids and sick nurses. The matrons were to have oversight of all the women and children and reported to the governors. The matron's duties included the supervision of laundry, bedding, stocktaking, cleaning, the appearance of the keepers and night rounds. The keepers were to be virtuous and they were responsible for observations, management, cleanliness, occupation, chastity, order at night, reporting faults and punishments (Russell 1997).

Generally the male keepers were recruited from the class of farm servants fresh from the country and the females predominantly from the class of domestic servants. They were the unemployed of other occupations. If they possessed physical strength, and a tolerable reputation for sobriety, it was enough. They entered the occupation altogether ignorant of what constituted insanity but with the idea that their charges were no longer capable of reasoning or feeling and that in order to manage, it was necessary to terrify and coerce them. The insane were held to be insensible to variations of temperature hence their confinement, usually chained, in unwarmed rooms and cellars. Treatment, if given, was confined to bleedings, purgatives or emetics. Chains, belts, bars, locks, keys, stocks, cribs secured with chains, fetters and chains, irregular meals, want of exercise, abusive words, contemptuous names, blows with the fist or straps or keys formed an almost daily part of their lives. At the same time the inmates were expected to do domestic work, general maintenance and gardening. The social status of the keepers was no more than that of domestic servants and they were subjected to as much discipline and surveillance as were their charges (O'Donaghue 1914).

In 1601 the Poor Law Act focused attention on the poor, the aged, the disabled, the idiot and the lunatic and gave magistrates and other county justices the authority to oversee their well-being (Allderidge 1979). These people were then placed in the custody of keepers and beadles in bridewells and madhouses.

PHYSICIANS AND THE 'TRADE IN LUNACY'

The physicians played no part in the early confinement but became an essential figure from the late 17th and the 18th centuries. By the end of the 18th century the physician had consolidated confinement into a medical space, with medical practice being for a long time no more than a complement to the old rites of order, authority, discipline and punishment.

Alongside these developments were the private madhouses and the madhouse trade, called the 'trade in lunacy', which grew in all parts of the country (Parry-Jones 1972). One of the origins of this madhouse system for pauper lunatics was the practice of boarding out the insane at the expense of the parish in private dwelling houses, which then acquired the description of madhouses. Another was the demand on the part of the upper classes for some system of private care, which would relieve them of the burden of their unmanageable relatives. Besides these private institutions run for profit, there were a number of charitable institutions set up to provide for the poor but respectable classes (Jones 1955).

These private madhouses had a variety of persons in charge: doctors, clergymen, quacks and laymen. The proprietor often acted as superintendent but these positions could be combined or held by separate individuals. The term keeper was often used to denote both master of the madhouse and a person attending the insane.

The assumption of medical responsibility for the insane, however, was a slow process, particularly in private madhouses. The selection of the Reverend Dr Francis Wills to treat King George III in 1788 was therefore an event of considerable importance in the history of medical madhouse proprietors and doctors of the insane. It brought some professional respectability to the 'trade in lunacy' and demonstrated that the treatment of insanity required the special skills and experience not necessarily possessed by the most eminent physicians of the day (Hunter and Macalpine 1963). Wills made an important contribution by propagating the notion that insanity was curable, thereby removing the excuses for neglect which therapeutic pessimism had fostered for centuries.

There was at this time a fight for the lucrative trade in lunacy. The medical men who owned and ran most of the madhouses wanted to outlaw the lay madhouse keepers. Many physicians stated openly that the treatment was superior in madhouses kept by medical men. They pictured lay keepers as ignorant, illiterate and of low integrity. Burrows (1828) stated that in madhouses kept by non-medical keepers, all that was offered was custody while those houses kept by doctors offered cure. He gave his views in evidence to the 1828 Select Committee of the House of Lords and his remarks reflected the view that lay proprietors were more likely to be corrupt and avaricious than medically trained proprietors. By 1860 the official policy as stated by the Commissioners was not to issue new licences other than to medical proprietors. The high demand for private madhouse accommodation resulted in many single medical people owning a number of madhouses but residing in none, instead delegating responsibilities to superintendents, keepers, servants and attendants.

The role and nature of the duties of the madhouse attendant or keeper changed considerably with the development of the private madhouse system. Walk (1954, 1961) has drawn attention to the praiseworthy work of attendants in the early to mid-19th century, when attendants were employed in madhouses and hospitals which housed paupers and private lunatics and in madhouses for the wealthy. Walk (1961) has argued that attendants were involved in the move from custodial duties and the uses of mechanical restraint to employing the technique of moral restraint developed by Tuke at the York Retreat.

DEVELOPMENT OF THE ASYLUM SYSTEM

The attendants were the category of workers which replaced the keepers and saw the development of the asylum system. Their roles and functions were governed by rule books which dictated all their relationships with the inmates and the institution. The rules dictated that discipline was seen as the first duty of attendants. This discipline, with its close association with surveillance, related to three aspects of the attendants' work. First, it dictated the attendants' duty to the institution and their colleagues. Second, it covered the duties to inmates. Third, it demanded behaviour as an example; that is, the attendants were required to set an example of industry, order, cleanliness and obedience. This discipline was associated also with the utilization of the inmates' labour and the latter part of the 19th century saw rapid development in industries within asylum/hospital buildings and grounds. While some attendants were confined to tending debilitated inmates or surveillance of those taking exercises on airing, courts, others spent much time supervising the work of inmates. Security occupied most of the rules and regulations, particularly with regard to the care of keys, tools and cutlery. Given the low wages, long hours and poor conditions, the managers of hospitals/asylums set fairly modest ideals for recruitment (Duncan 1809, Burdette 1891, O'Donaghue 1914).

The principle of moral restraint that was put forward by Tuke (1813) argued that the distraction of the inmates' minds was a result of their blind surrender to desires and an incapacity to control passions. Therefore insanity could be corrected by a regime to establish self-discipline. Tuke sought to reproduce in the York Retreat the intimacy of family relations, with the insane as dependent children and himself as an authoritarian patriarch.

Force and mechanical restraint were to be used only as a last resort. The main aim of the moral treatment was assisting the insane to control themselves, the theory being that a less coercive form of control would better lead to the internalization of the principle of self-control. Conolly (1856) argued that the pursuit of moral principles depended on the qualities of those caring for the inmates, the attendants. Since the principle of non-restraint was to exclude all hurtful excitement from a brain already disposed to excitement, it was said that the physician who understood the non-restraint system knew that the attendants were his most essential instrument.

Browne (1837), in his book *What Asylums Were, Are and Ought to Be*, had called for some system of instruction for attendants. However, it was not until between 1842 and 1844 that Sir Alexander Morrison gave the first-known set of lectures to attendants at the Surrey asylum. This was followed in 1854 by a course of 30 lectures given to attendants and doctors by Browne at the Chirchton Royal Hospital.

In 1871, Henry Maudsley proposed that the Medico-Psychological Association should set up a registry of good attendants but he did not attempt to link this with any form of training. The development of training enabled attendants to establish themselves as carers of the insane and at the same time gain mobility and enhanced promotion prospects. Examination papers were set centrally by the Medico-Psychological Association, with the conduct of the examination and the marking of the papers left to the institution's medical superintendent and an external assessor.

In 1885 the Medico-Psychological Association published a *Handbook for Attendants on the Insane* (Campbell-Clark *et al.* 1885). The book was published by a committee of Scottish members of the Medico-Psychological Association and consisted of a thin volume of 64 pages. It was prepared in the hope of helping attendants on the insane to understand better the work in which they were engaged. It sought to provide information on the body and mind in health and disease, instructions on the management of the illnesses and rules to enable them to function with intelligence and watchfulness. It was intended that the instructions should help attendants to carry out the orders of the physician, while emphasizing that the contents of the book cannot override the special rules of any institution or special orders relating to individual cases.

The text was divided into the following chapters: the body, its general functions and disorders, the nursing of the sick, mind and its disorders, the care of the insane, and the general duties of the attendants. The book, Nolan (1993) stated, can be regarded as a significant advance in the progress of mental nursing because it represented a shift from the oral tradition through which the attendant's work was described to a written one.

It is clear from the contents of the handbook that the medical understanding of treatment of the insane was given priority. By 1891 the Medico-Psychological Association had acquired the prefix 'Royal'. It extended the training of attendants to three years with control over the content of training remaining with doctors. The syllabus was dominated by the basic sciences of anatomy, physiology and neurology. At this time the attendants, supported by some members of the Royal Medico-Psychological Association, started the Asylum Workers' Union, with the aim of promoting the interests and status of attendants and others engaged in the care of the insane.

The middle of the 19th century saw the development of the asylum system in institutions designed to control, care for and treat the insane. The asylums did not hold out the promise of cure but instead became establishments which exercised control. As they increased in size, the attendants maintained harsh regimes which included mechanical, chemical and dietary restraints. There was also a strong emphasis on the orderly management of the attendants and the insane. The 1845 Lunatics Act had some humanitarian aspects to it. The Act asked for the blurring of the distinction between mental and physical disorders, the protection of the insane against illegal detention and for the involvement of social workers.

A main achievement of this period was in the area of illegal detention. The Lunatics' Friend Society was founded by Luke James Hansard, the son of the original printer of the House of Commons. Along with Lord Ashley and his group of parliamentary reformers, he petitioned Parliament and achieved the protection of the British subject from unjust confinement on grounds of mental derangement (Jones 1972).

The 1890 Lunacy Act was developed in a social climate which had become critical of the services available for the insane. The Act stated that mechanical restraint instruments and appliances was only to be used for the purposes of surgical or medical treatment or to prevent patients injuring themselves or fellow patients. A medical certificate was necessary for each instance of restraint and a report book had to be kept; all such records were to be sent to the Commissioners in Lunacy once every quarter. The use of mechanical restraint and instruments had made the attendants' job much easier. Restraints were applied to the melancholic, the maniac or the violent patient. Suicidal patients did not have to be watched and night attendance was avoided because they were strapped to their beds. Alongside these mechanical restraints was the use of water, air and electricity.

Improvements in the treatment of the insane under this Act were encouraged by the initiatives in training. Male and female attendants were achieving the Royal Medico-Psychological Association certificate, with most of the training offered by the doctors, which included massage and first aid.

According to Strahan (1986), the attendants were being made aware of the broader medical context of psychiatry and the part they had to play. Attendants' training was considered to be inferior to general nursing training and when attempts were made to get the Royal British Nursing Association to recognize the Royal Medico-Psychological Association qualification, there was opposition. However, in 1895 the resolution was adopted and moves began to bring mental nursing in line with other kinds of nursing. This was finally sealed by the Nurses' Registration Act for England, Scotland and Wales 1919. However, it was not until 1943 that the Royal College of Nursing accepted mental nurses by virtue of mental nurses being additionally qualified as general nurses. By 1951 training for mental nurses had passed entirely into the hands of the General Nursing Council.

DEVELOPMENT OF MODERN MENTAL HEALTH NURSING

The Mental Treatment Act 1930 was passed within a climate of belief that viewing mental illness as being similar to physical illness would minimise the stigma of mental illness. This physical illness approach contributed to the decision by Parliament to pass an Act which placed the treatment, care and control of the mentally ill with doctors. Attempts to cure mental illness saw the vigorous use of insulin therapy, electroconvulsive therapy, surgery and drug therapy. This clinical somatic approach brought changes in the training and expected skills of the mental nurse. They were expected to be skilled in the following treatments: sedation, relaxation, insulin therapy, malaria and sulphosin therapy, diet and vitamin therapy, endocrine and drug therapies, operating interventions, rehabilitation, psychotherapy, massage and hydrotherapy.

However, along with these mainly physical interventions, the mental nurse still entertained patients and shared in domestic chores such as floor polishing. They were responsible for farm work, industrial work and overall surveillance. At the same time they were the main functionaries through which custody and control involving straitjackets, padded cells and force feeding took place. Other developments at this time included occupational therapy, psychology and social work. The asylums were now rechristened mental hospitals and the inmates referred to as patients and clinics for mental disorders were associated with general hospitals and medical schools.

The 1959 Mental Health Act came into force with mental nurses being involved with physical restraint and the maintenance of institutional life. At the same time the new emphasis on community care contributed to the development of community psychiatric nursing. This mixed background gave rise to the extension of the psychiatric nurse's role into working outside the hospital caring for discharged patients in their homes, at health centres and in outpatients departments.

The hospitals which pioneered the development of community psychiatric nursing were Warlingham Park in Croydon in 1954 and Moorhaven in Devon in 1957. The role and function of psychiatric nurse in the community embraced the following:

- helping the family and other carers with the management of the patient
- being the link between the patient and the hospital so that the patient could be readmitted quickly if there is a relapse or a breakdown in care
- the giving of continuous care to all categories of patients
- the maintenance of the patients' prescriptions
- the recognition of side effects and taking appropriate action
- a preventive role by going to the aid of patients whose illness does not require treatment in a clinic or a hospital and the giving of advice, support and supervision.

Hunter (1956) has suggested that the introduction of psychotropic drugs resulted in the deskilling of the mental nurses. Studies were undertaken to examine the work, role and function of the mental nurse. For example, Oppenheim and Erman (1955) examined the role and training of mental nursing and this was followed by research by Maddox (1957) and John (1961). All these studies reported the complex activities involved in mental health work, the shortage of resources and the difficulties experienced in recruiting suitable candidates.

The Salmon Report (DHSS 1966) on nursing management structure created the new role of nursing officer. The nursing officer had responsibility for planning and overseeing clinical supervision, management and personnel work.

This new structure saw an increase in mobility and competitiveness amongst nursing staff but sadly it was never evaluated and therefore the nursing officer's contributions can only be anecdotal.

Throughout the 1960s the activities in mental hospitals became a public concern, with the public asking questions about conditions in these institutions. At the same time staff, despairing of changing the system from within, called upon outsiders for help. Letters were written to newspapers and Robb (1967) published *Sans Everything: a case to answer*. This book contributed to a closer look being taken at the care and treatment given to vulnerable groups such as the elderly, children, and mentally ill and the mentally handicapped. Many inquiries and reports followed and these reports, with comments, were published in Martin (1984). The inquiries found cruelty to patients and pilfering of their food and indifference to such malpractice on the part of the senior nurse and medical management.

The 1983 Mental Health Act moved the approaches to care and treatment into the rights arena which, while not reducing the clinical-somatic approach, attempted to increase the civil rights of patients. Social workers were now to be more involved in admission procedures and the Mental Health Review Tribunal was required to respond more rapidly. A new body, the Mental Health Act Commission, was established to ensure good practice and to make sure that the procedures for consent to treatment and second opinion were followed.

Mental nurses have remained central to the running of hospital wards and only a minority have become involved in community care. The clinical-somatic approach to care has resulted in most of the mental nurses' functions being concentrated on maintaining medication. However, these same changes also made possible the development of new mental nursing skills such as group work, therapeutic community skills, counselling skills and psychotherapy skills. The result is that mental nurses are once again emphasizing their role in developing interpersonal therapeutic relationships with patients.

The Jay Report (DHSS 1979) looked critically at the work of mental handicap nursing. Following this report, the Mental Nurse Committee of the General Nursing Council decided to change the mental nurse training syllabus, in an attempt to preempt any of the Jay Report findings being applied to mental nursing. The new syllabus emphasized the acquisition of interpersonal skills, signalling the end of institutional training and an assertion of professional independence. It also showed that mental nurses were beginning to adopt social and psychological models, to favour the title therapist and to see themselves as the centre of the therapeutic process. The syllabus also presented mental nursing as essentially different from general nursing. However, this position was radically undermined a decade later with the introduction of the Project 2000 training which emphasized similarities between all nursing, the abolition of direct entry and the institution of a Common Foundation Programme.

Throughout the history of mental nursing the wishes of superintendents and doctors, along with legislation, have contributed to changes in the role and function of mental nurses who left behind some of their interpersonal social skills of care and adopted a clinical-somatic approach to care. This approach, although useful, cannot provide for all the needs of the mentally ill person. However, since the Acts of 1959 and 1983 mental nurses have been trying to regain the social aspects of care within their work. Mental health legislation has contributed greatly to major changes in the social treatment and care of mental illness. First, there was the rise of the asylum and the capture of that domain by the medical men. Second came an extension of the concept of mental illness, along with control and surveillance within and without the asylums and madhouses, and the development of new therapies and professions, notably social work, occupational therapy, psychology and psychoanalysis. The integration of the legal and the medical emphasized the power of psychiatry as a method of defining and regulating social behaviour.

At the start of the new millennium mental nurses are trying to deal with the complexities of their roles and functions. These roles embrace mental health and professional legal statutes, the medical, social and psychological aspects of care and treatment and the social control realities of their work. Therefore the mental nurse's roles and functions embrace the knowledge and skills associated with the provision of psychosocial therapeutic care where people learn to modify their antisocial behaviour through experiencing different socialisation activities. This type of intervention draws heavily on the nurse–patient relationship where the nurse is working *with* patients rather than *for* them (Skellern 1957). The use of behaviour therapy was established at the Maudsley Hospital in 1957. Here the mental nurse, under medical supervision, achieved a successful advanced clinical role within the hospital and in primary care. The nurse recruited to this work adopted a more scientific and research-oriented approach to care and treatment.

Other interventions were also being developed in psychodynamic methods and nurses trained as psychotherapists, cognitive therapists and counsellors. While all these trainings and interventions were taking place the role and function of the community psychiatric nurse continued to develop and to respond to the needs of society, particularly in the light of limited resources and public fears about the behaviour of mentally ill people in the community. This has led to an increasing policy emphasis on the need for community mental health nurses to prioritize those with 'severe and enduring' mental health problems (DoH 1996) who are deemed to be either a risk to themselves or others or to require control and surveillance to maintain their care and treatment programmes. This surveillance and control role is clear in the Mental Health Patients in the Community Act 1995 (DoH 1995). This development of supervised aftercare may also be regarded as in some way linked to a return of the dominance of the medical somatic approach to the care and treatment of the mentally ill.

THE FUTURE

Within the framework of the limitations on their work imposed by legislation, professional ideologies, limited resources and public attitudes, it is clear from the activities of mental nurses that they have some capacity to take forward a radical agenda for mental health service provision.

The work of mental nurses must be considered as a departure from adult (general) nursing. Perhaps a new occupational group is required for the future. However, even if the workers for the mentally ill remain within the category of nursing, they should be trained to challenge the contradiction in psychiatry whereby it is simultaneously a regulatory social apparatus and a system of treatment and care. Such workers would lend a new emphasis to the need to empower and protect the rights of the person deemed to be mentally ill. In so doing, they would draw on the ideas of Karl Marx who saw the economic relationships of capitalism as having consequences for social relationships through the process of alienation. They would address the need to work with people at the community level, to know about unemployment, poor housing, low wages and the health of the environment, along with the social, health, welfare and educational services which exist. As a more political group of health workers, they could become involved in the political process through joining with user groups to ask for more resources and better facilities to provide care. To ask survivors, were your rights infringed by the mental health services and how? To ask users and carers, how can the mental health services ensure that rights are respected and not abused?

In order to take on this role, mental nurses would need a different type of education, one with more emphasis on the social sciences, counselling, mental health promotion, philosophy and law, along with specialist medical and psychiatric knowledge.

These political activities of the new mental nurse might take place at both the national and the local level and would include the interrogation of medical judgements and treatments for their effectiveness and safety and especially the need for more information about the side effects of prescribed drugs and the use of electroconvulsive therapy. The issues around social divisions, patriarchy, class and racism which result in life problems and mental distress would be addressed. In so doing, exclusion and oppression would be examined and confronted.

Of great importance would be the need to develop a strong sense of accountability as a prerequisite for working with people. It would involve a commitment to respond to questions, challenges and the requests of users and would be rooted in a belief that professional activity is intended to aid the user. Users would also be empowered to emphasize more their role in educating service providers, including social workers, psychiatrists and mental nurses, which could lead to a more positive collaborative working environment.

Taking up the challenge of developing these possible new ways of working will not be easy. The mental nurse's desire for power will still be there, the political, economic, social and medical realities will be present and exerting their influences. However, recent government publications look closely at how the role of the mental health nurse can be developed in conjunction with users and carers in order to provide a service which meets closely the needs of all concerned in the process of nursing, whether in the institution or in the community.

REFERENCES

Allderidge, P. (1979 Hospitals, Madhouses and Asylums: cycles in the care of the insane. *British Journal of Psychiatry* **134**: 321–334.

Browne, W.A.F. (1937) *What Asylums Were, Are and Ought to Be.* Adam Charles, Edinburgh.

Burdette, H.C. (1891) *Hospitals and Asylums of the World: their origin, history, construction, administration, management and legislation.* Churchill, London.

Burrows, G.M. (1828) *Commentaries on the Causes of Insanity.* Underwood, London.

Campbell-Clark, A., MacIver-Campbell, C., Turnbull, A.R. and Urquhart, A.R. (1885) *Handbook for Attendants on the Insane.* Ballière Tindall, London.

Conolly, J. (1856) *The Treatment of the Insane without Mechanical Restraint.* Smith Elder, London.

DHSS (1966) *The Report of the Committee on Senior Nurse Staffing Structure (The Salmon Report).* HMSO, London.

DHSS (1979) *Report of the Committee of Enquiry into Mental Handicap Nursing (The Jay Report).* HMSO, London.

DoH (1995) *The Mental Health Patients in the Community Act.* HMSO, London.

DoH (1996) *The Spectrum of Care: local services for people with mental health problems.* HMSO, London.

Duncan, A. (1809). *Observations on the Structure of Hospitals for the Treatment of Lunatics.* Ballantyre, Edinburgh.

Edwards, A.H. (1975) *Mental Health Services.* Shaw, London.

Hunter, R. (1956) The rise and fall of mental nursing in the mental hospital. *Lancet* **July 14**: 98–99.

Hunter, R. and Macalpine, L. (1963) *Three Hundred Years of Psychiatry 1535–1860.* Castle Publishing, New York.

John, A. (1961) *A Study of the Psychiatric Nurse.* E.&S. Livingstone, Edinburgh.

Jones, K. (1955) *Lunacy, Law and Conscience 1744–1845.* Routledge and Kegan Paul, London.

Jones, K. (1972) *A History of Mental Health Services.* Routledge and Kegan Paul, London.

Maddox, H. (1957) The work of the mental nurse. *Nursing Mirror* **105**: 189–191.

Martin, J.P. (1984) *Hospitals in Trouble.* Basil Blackwell, London.

Nolan, P. (1993) *A History of Mental Health Nursing.* Chapman and Hall, London.

O'Donaghue, E.C. (1914) *The Story of Bethlem Hospital from its Foundation in 1247.* T. Fisher Unwin, London.

Oppenheim, A.M. and Erman, B. (1955) *The Function and Training of the Mental Nurse.* Chapman and Hall, London.

Parry-Jones, P. (1972) *The Trade in Lunacy.* Routledge and Kegan Paul, London.

Robb, B. (ed.) (1967) *Sans Everything: a case to answer.* Nelson, London.

Russell, D. (1997) *Scenes From Bedlam.* Baillière Tindall, London.

Skellern, E. (1957) From custodial to therapeutic care. *Nursing Times* **53**(8): 209–211, 220–221.

Strahan, S.A.K. (1986) Can the medical spirit be kept up in asylums for the insane? *Journal of Mental Science* **32**: 344.

Tuke, S. (1813) *Description of Retreat.* W. Darton, London.

Walk, A. (1954) Some aspects of the moral treatment of the insane up to 1854. *Journal of Mental Science* **100**: 807–837.

Walk, A. (1961). The history of mental nursing. *Journal of Mental Science* **107**: 1–17.

2 THE NURSE AS ASSESSOR

Stuart Donald, Rob Lancaster, Sheila Forster

OBJECTIVES

After reading this chapter, you should be able to:

- understand the purpose of assessment in mental health nursing
- identify the context in which the assessment of the client takes place with particular reference to recent policy developments in mental health services, including the Care Programme Approach
- describe the interviewing skills required by the nurse assessor
- explain the significance of the admission profile, history taking and the examination of the client's mental state at the point of assessment
- discuss various approaches to data collection and their applicability to various situations
- demonstrate the importance of the nurse's role in assessing risk, notably in terms of the need to provide safe, sound and secure services for people suffering with severe and enduring mental illnesses.

INTRODUCTION

This chapter introduces a number of key ideas about assessment in mental health nursing. The purpose of assessment and the context in which it will take place is described. An overview of the Care Programme Approach and related policy initiatives will be provided and their implications for mental health nursing, and the process of assessment in particular, will be considered. Basic clinical risk assessment is an area in which mental health nurses will need to be increasingly proficient.

Health care is an increasingly politicized and publicly exposed arena and no practitioner can ignore this and this raises a number of points for assessment in clinical practice. The critique of the community mental health care policy has led to a greater emphasis on the supervision of mentally disordered people (Lingham *et al.* 1997, Ritchie *et al.* 1994). Mental health nurses need to understand the significance of accurate assessment as part of the process of assisting people with severe mental illnesses to live in the community and to help prevent people slipping through the net of care. As resources need to become increasingly targeted, assessment will be used to determine eligibility for services. The internal market has led to the 'commodification' of health care and mental health nursing has become a health care product which a primary care group may or may not want to commission. Accordingly, the quality of assessment has become more open to scrutiny and the focus on time-limited interventions as a means of cost containment has become tighter. There is a growing emphasis on evidence-based approaches to treatment which mental health nurses need to understand and adopt.

Overall, the last two decades have seen a huge increase in interest in the concept of assessment. Whilst it would be foolish to appear dismissive about the necessity of accurate assessment, it could be argued that there has been something of an overvaluation of the topic. In the nursing world this was initiated in the idea of nursing as a process which was met with resistance when introduced often in a mandatory fashion. Nursing along with other professions has become more and more preoccupied with assessment formats and documen-tation. There are risks that endless working groups may be convened within services to consider the latest assessment themes often with no accompanying attention to the importance of outcome. The search for the best assessment tool has become like the pursuit of the Holy Grail, leading to the underestimation of the role of interpersonal skills and relationship development.

THE PURPOSE OF ASSESSMENT

The purpose of assessment in mental health nursing is to define the service user's mental health status and needs. This will require the collection and organization of valid information about the problems that the service user is seeking help for. As far as possible this should be a collaborative process between the service user, the mental health nurse and, where relevant, the views of other professionals and carers. Assessment should be 'needs led' as far as practicable as opposed to being service led (Onyett 1992, p 116), i.e. people are not fitted into available services but rather services are designed to meet the needs of people. Nevertheless, a key aim of assessment must be to identify whether a person has been referred to the right service and would not receive more appropriate help elsewhere. An accurate assessment will form the basis of effective care and treatment planning.

In addition to defining the service user's needs, the assessment should also identify the individual's personal strengths or resources which can be mobilized. The mental health nurse's approach should be comprehensive or holistic in that it takes account of the range of relevant dimensions within the service user's life, e.g., accommodation, finances, occupation, rather than focusing solely upon the symptoms of mental disorder. It should recognize the interrelationship of these dimensions and how they affect the life of the individual. Whereas the Care Programme Approach (CPA) has been criticized for advocating a somewhat reductionist attitude in defining need as either 'social' or 'health care' in nature (Huxley 1990), a valid term to describe a desired style of assessment would be 'biopsychosocial'.

Assessment should take account of immediate, medium and long-term needs and increasingly mental health nurses are required to contribute to the assessment of risk. An effective assessment is not merely a list of disparate areas of need to be met but should produce a framework which allows relevant goal setting. Furthermore, the assessment should generate a hierarchy of needs which will inform the process of delivering care. In other words, assessment is but one step in an integrated system of organizing care and treatment. Such a system may be illustrated by a sequence, such as in the care management cycle of:

- case finding
- assessment
- care planning
- implementation
- evaluation and review
- case closure (see Onyett 1992, pp. 29–31).

ASSESSMENT AND REASSESSMENT

Assessment should not be seen as a 'one-shot' process but as something which is continuous and dynamic in nature. At each contact with the service user, the mental health nurse should be assessing how the person is doing. In addition to this form of ongoing assessment, there should be specific milestones at which care and treatment are formally reviewed, which may lead to a reassessment. This may be particularly relevant at times such as before discharge from hospital. Review and reassessment form part of the sequence described above and local services will specify the frequency of review within CPA procedures.

PRINCIPLES OF THE CARE PROGRAMME APPROACH

Mental health care should be organized within the context of the CPA (DoH 1990) which remains the cornerstone of the government's mental health policy and is intended to ensure 'that all patients are assessed and that no one who might be vulnerable is missed' (DoH 1994). This requires a systematic assessment of the health and social care needs of a person who has been referred to the 'specialist mental health services'. A primary aim of the CPA is to improve the delivery of care to people with severe mental illness (DoH 1994). An integral part of the CPA is the identification of a 'key worker' who will work with the service user and carer to assess needs, develop and implement a care plan. Mental health nurses working in community settings will undertake the role of CPA key worker which carries a range of coordination and leadership tasks.

More recent guidance about CPA has recommended the adoption of tiering which enables a differentiation of people referred to services (DoH 1994). Those people using services who have enduring mental illnesses and accompanying complex needs will be classified in a higher tier and will receive a 'complex or multidisciplinary CPA'. This will involve a high level of formality in developing the assessment and accompanying care plans. The CPA plan should be seen as the overall or agreed single plan (DoH 1994) for the individual and the inputs of the various participants should contribute to this plan:

- nursing plan
- OT plan
- medical plan
- social care plan.

Mental health nurses acting as hospital key workers/primary nurses or as CPA key workers will need to ensure that all relevant players contribute to the assessment which should cover all relevant dimensions of the service user's life. In the CPA key worker role, the nurse is instrumental in identifying a range of assessment requirements, some of which may be beyond the nurse's own expertise. In addition to the disruption caused by mental illness, many service users with severe and enduring mental illnesses, particularly schizophrenia, will be disadvantaged by 'secondary impairment' (Stein and Test 1980). This will result in a form of disability characterized by difficulty coping with activities of daily living that the majority of people take for granted such as coping with public transport, shopping, cooking, finding accommodation and dealing with officialdom. Specialist assessments from workers such as occupational therapists, social workers and benefits advisors must be sought. These will need to be aggregated into an overall care plan which is relevant, comprehensible and acceptable to service users.

RISK ASSESSMENT

Increasingly mental health nurses need to understand the importance of risk assessment and to be proficient in this area. Assessing risk should be incorporated within the overall assessment of an individual's needs rather than be approached as a separate and compartmentalized area for assessment. The DoH circular *Guidance on the Discharge of Mentally Disordered People and Their Continuing Care in the Community* offers practitioners some important pointers about how to assess risk. There are four subject areas that require assessment: the risk of self-harm, harm to others or dangerousness, self-neglect and serious exploitation. Risk assessment is an inexact science (DoH 1995) and inevitably different practitioners will regard the existence or extent of risk in varying ways. According to the experience and work context of each practitioner, they will have their own threshold at which risk will be regarded as a problem. Individual teams and departments need to develop their own policies and a common vocabulary to describe risk.

Risk is generally classified as low, medium or high depending upon the probability that an adverse incident will occur and the severity of the consequences of that incident. Some approaches attempt to quantify risk by rating the probability and severity numerically and multiplying these two factors to generate a composite score.

Probability $(0-5)$ × Severity $(0-5)$ = Risk rating

Where there is evidence of risk, e.g. imminent self-harm, an action plan must be developed following locally agreed protocols. Suggestion of medium risk or above should trigger a multidisciplinary assessment and the nurse must appraise the urgency with which this should take place.

The ability to undertake risk assessment competently and confidently will come with training and experience. Managers should ensure that junior and inexperienced staff are not expected to undertake assessments of new referrals or of people with histories of risk behaviour.

The process of assessing risk may place nurses in conflict with people using services. The first problematic area concerns the style of assessment. Information about risk factors should be ascertained during the assessment process. This will mean asking explicit questions about risk including gauging both the degree of *ideation* and *intentionality* about a possible adverse event. In many situations, e.g. impatient psychiatry, a history will be taken on admission which identifies risk behaviours and past events which needs to be shared within the multidisciplinary as well as the nursing team. However, in community settings the nurse may be the first contact with the service. A tension may exist between adopting a needs-led approach and assessing and managing risk. This may be especially evident in situations where people experience acute distress and are unable to manage their own behaviour and may even require restraint, detention and compulsory treatment. Such approaches need to operate within a context where attitudes do not become defensive, care plans do not reduce all interventions to the lowest common denominator and services drift into a paternalistic approach.

Concern over the community mental health-care policy has led to a focus upon the importance of assessing risk, particularly at the predischarge stage. This emphasis is intended to avoid people 'slipping through the net of care'.

ASSESSMENT IN A CHANGING CLIMATE

A new approach is emerging within mental health services based upon the concept of supervision of people who pose a risk to themselves or to others. The relationship of this type of supervision to assessment needs to be understood, as does the wider political and public thinking about mental health care. The identification and management of risk is a central component of this form of supervision. Mental health nurses should understand the significance of *prodromal* signs in the people they are working with and will identify *relapse indicators* and develop *contingency arrangements* in care plans.

The concept of supervising people with mental health problems has led to the prioritization of resources upon the seriously mentally ill. Such prioritization is primarily linked to anxiety about the community mental health-care policy in the UK. Other supporting factors include the accompanying debates about the remit of health-care provision in UK, what are to be provided as core services and the growing focus on evidence-based approaches. The concept of supervision inevitably requires that the nurse assesses from the perspective of calculating, minimizing risk and curbing behavioural excesses. The significance of supervision is increasingly illustrated through the terminology used in policy and legislation, e.g. the supervision register and the supervised discharge amendment (Section 25a).

The mental health nurse plays a major part in the execution of the present community mental health-care policy. This policy is based upon certain ideological and legislative principles which have arguably outlived their sell-by date. As long ago as 1986, Rose argued that the 1983 mental health legislation was based upon flawed concepts of rights and libertarian ideologies that were not relevant to the UK scene. Rose criticized many aspects of the American experience of deinstitutionalization which had led to patients 'dying with their rights on'. A significant ideological shift has emerged during the past decade from the libertarian principles underpinning the 1983 Mental Health Act to a greater concern with public safety. Concern over mental health policy led to the famous statement by a previous Secretary of State for Health, Virginia Bottomley, that 'the pendulum has swung too far' and the subsequent publication of the 'Ten Point Plan' which heralded the 1995 Amendment to the Mental Patients in the Community Act and the earlier introduction of psychiatric supervision registers (Burns 1994).

The community mental health-care policy has attracted consistent media attention and growing criticism. It is a policy about which the previous government became increasingly ambivalent and sensitive to criticism and from which the present government has explicitly sought to distance itself (Dobson 1998) by proposing a fundamental review of existing policy and legislation. Homicides by mentally disordered people (by far outstripped by the number of suicides) have attracted mounting scrutiny and a number of services have been examined in painful detail when a disaster has occurred (see Lingham et al. 1996, Ritchie et al. 1994).

Reports into community care 'failures' or breakdowns have highlighted two critical areas: failure to assess risk satisfactorily and failures of communication between professionals and agencies. The expectation has been expressed that assessment can identify those people most at risk who will then be treated as a priority group. It is recognized that risk assessment is an inexact science and some have argued that homicides by people with mental illnesses are a rare phenomenon and cannot be anticipated. Nevertheless, there is a firm public and managerial expectation that all the mental health professionals should perform better and are seen to perform better when it comes to preventing major incidents. Professionals themselves may feel increasingly at risk of public censure if people in their care commit dangerous acts or harm themselves. Accordingly there is a greater level of exposure to risk arising from the decisions made about the clinical management of the most vulnerable people using services. Senior clinical staff and managers are developing an anticipatory sense of how their decisions would appear in the inquiry which will follow any major incident.

The crucial point for mental health nurses is to ensure that they understand the climate in which they operate, the need to identify both risk and relapse indicators and how to initiate necessary action.

THE CONTEXT OF ASSESSMENT

Assessment does not take place in a vacuum. As shown in the previous section, it is rarely a politically or ideologically free activity. There are certain contextual issues involved that need to be both understood and anticipated by the mental health nurse. Those themes covered below are undoubtedly not the end of the story but it is hoped that they will provide an illustration.

Multidisciplinary assessment

To achieve a full assessment of an individual's need, the mental health nurse will have to work closely with other professionals who have a contribution to make to the overall care plan. This will be particularly necessary when people present with complex needs which may require a range of interventions. Each person's assessment will need to be available to all relevant professionals and collectively cover the crucial areas of need for the service user. The logical means of organizing multidisciplinary inputs will be through the effective use of the CPA. The nurse needs to recognize the contribution that others can make and be confident about working alongside other professionals.

Bias, pitfalls and style

Bias must be guarded against in the assessment process. Bias can manifest itself in two ways. Whilst it must be accepted that assessment never takes place in a value-free setting, the mental health nurse should consciously guard against approaching assessment from a single theoretical perspective. For example, the nurse with a behavioural/cognitive orientation may assess people within that framework. This could disadvantage the client who may see his problems in a different way. It is critical for the nurse to ensure that a shared perspective is developed during the assessment and that the process is not unduly led by the professional. This is a further illustration of the hazards of fitting people to services rather than vice versa.

The second pitfall can occur when assessing the client whose history precedes him. People who have displayed episodes of violent behaviour may become 'sensationalized' within services and great skill will be required to avoid adopting a defensive perception. This is not to deny that some people with mental health problems do commit acts of violence and when particularly unwell may do so again. In fact, this point is well argued in various reports: 'the only decent predictor of future behaviour is past behaviour' (Ritchie *et al.* 1994). Nevertheless, accurate assessment, particularly of risk, needs to be as objective as possible. Additionally, accounts of previous incidents need to be understood within the context in which they occurred.

A further difficulty revolves around the use of assessment documentation. As suggested in the introduction, there has been a growing emphasis on this area. There are sound and clear reasons for accurate documentation covering assessment as well as other areas of practice. In addition to ethical and legal considerations, there is a demand for greater transparency which has been driven to an extent by the Access to Information Act (DoH 1991). Furthermore, the multidisciplinary context requires that each profession's documentation must be accessible and coherent to all involved in an individual's care and treatment. However, overemphasis upon documentation may jeopardize the development of a meaningful interpersonal relationship between the nurse and service user.

Barker (1997) has emphasized the importance of this therapeutic relationship and has underlined a distinction between the fields of nursing and psychiatry. The former seeks to focus on a person's *experience* of a mental illness such as schizophrenia, whereas the latter concentrates on the person's mental illness (or absence of it). This distinction is not merely a semantic one. Naturally an assessment must establish the presence or absence of mental illness. There is a responsibility for all practitioners to target their efforts effectively. What must be avoided is a 'tick list' approach to assessment which fails to take account of the meaning of the mental disorder for the individual and how it disables that individual across a range of activities in their life. Both 'pussyfooting' around (Burnard 1991) with excessive smalltalk and resorting to a sledgehammer style of intrusive interrogation should be avoided. People may be referred to mental health services in a state of acute crisis and effective listening may be indicated (Truax and Carkhuff 1967).

The mental health nurse must learn to reconcile these apparently divergent demands. Accurate data must be obtained which provide a basis for care planning whilst avoiding insensitive questioning. Both sensitivity and directness will need to be employed which requires a considerable degree of flexibility and tenacity.

Time constraints

The workload of teams, service priorities and the 'commodification' of health care may require mental health nurses to work in a time-limited and highly focused way. Attention should be directed to the most pressing problems a person is presenting with. During the process of assessment the mental health nurse must identify those areas that are most critical for the service user. The fact that involvement will be time limited ought to be addressed in an explicit fashion with the patient/client during the assessment process so as to avoid misunderstandings later.

Separation of functions: purchasers/commissioners and providers

The NHS and Community Care Act 1990 introduced the separation of functions of purchasing and providers. More recently, this distinction has evolved into that of commissioning and provision in response to the new government's antipathy towards the notion of a 'market' within health and social services. Assessment may be linked to the commissioning function wherein there is no direct involvement of the person undertaking the assessment in the meeting of need identified.

This approach has been defined as service brokerage (Burns 1997) and in its most pure form relies upon a complete separation of the 'broker' from service delivery (DoH 1990). This approach is established within social services care management. It contrasts with the approaches more usually followed by health-care professionals who will assess and then attempt to meet identified need themselves. Now nurses may be involved in assessment of need with no accompanying expectation that they will meet that need. For instance, this will occur in the assessment of eligibility for services.

This separation of functions may prove problematic for nurses who have traditionally regarded assessment as an intrinsic part of engaging a person in the service. Additionally, this separation appears to contradict directly some of the arguments presented earlier where the importance of the interpersonal relationship has been described. However, dealing with contradiction is something that the mental health nurse must get used to!

Determining eligibility

Having argued that assessment should be needs led, mental health nurses practising in community settings will be concerned more and more with managing themselves as a resource. When assessing patients nurses must realize that there will always be limits on how much they can do and how much time is available. Priorities must be determined within departments and nurses must ensure that they adhere to these when assessing new referrals.

The mental health nurse may find herself assessing people to determine their eligibility for services. This will be especially applicable for community health nurses who will be accepting direct referrals from GPs and other members of the primary health-care team and who have also previously exercised great discretion over who to admit to a caseload. This requirement may prove difficult to meet as it challenges the universalist principle that the majority of health-care workers adhere to which is characterized by a belief that all people are entitled to receive services. Nurses will become accountable to colleagues, referrers and managers over their decisions about admissions to caseloads and assessment formats will need to demonstrate criteria to support such decisions.

At present the determination of eligibility may operate as an implicit rather than explicit process. Services having to focus resources upon those experiencing the most severe and enduring mental illnesses will achieve this by raising the 'threshold of morbidity' at which people will enter the service. Community mental health nurses will need to regard themselves as a financial resource and understand the principle of *opportunity costs* if resources are deployed in one way and not another.

Another area where front-line practitioners have to manage and deploy finite resources is in the management of psychiatric beds. Inner-city and more and more provincial services run with bed occupancy figures well in excess of 100%. This links to the earlier observation of the constraints of working within a risk-averse culture. The traditional way of managing psychiatric emergencies has been through hospital admission. Beds are blocked by the 'new long-stay population' and admitting acutely ill patients has become increasingly difficult. The closure of the Victorian asylums has led to a reduction in the number of beds available, particularly for those people suffering from enduring mental illnesses (Moore and Wolf 1999). Bed management is an example of where nurses may be acting as 'gatekeepers' and they will need to employ a widely agreed assessment tool to support this function. Due to the intense pressure upon psychiatric beds, many districts have sought to establish protocols to ensure that admission is reserved for those people who cannot be helped in other ways.

DEVELOPMENT OF THE MENTAL HEALTH NURSE ASSESSMENT

Although the act of assessing is by no means unfamiliar to the nurse much of its history has been characterized by relatively easy to obtain physiological indices (Savage 1991). Even as the discipline began to emerge from its subordinate position to the physician, the information gathered was still considered secondary to the medical assessment and was mainly used to furnish the doctor with additional baseline information from which a medical diagnosis could be made. However, the advances in our social, scientific and technological knowledge have helped develop nursing interventions and consequently led to a greater degree of sophistication being required of the assessment and greater skills of the nurse assessor. Even so it has been argued that assessment remains in its infancy (Barker 1997). Similarly concerned statements have termed it as the 'least proficient' of nursing roles in spite of an overwhelming agreement by nurses on its importance in nursing care.

As a consequence of this, mental health nurses have been left with a body of nursing knowledge on assessment that does not accurately reflect its importance, the result being that they have tended to establish their own individual ways of working (Morall 1995). Although this response is to be applauded as it has clearly demonstrated the resourcefulness of the discipline, it has also resulted in assessment practice being vulnerable to unacceptable degrees of bias and inconsistencies. Subsequently information gleaned at assessment by one nurse does not necessarily mirror information obtained by another nurse assessing the same person. Much of this can be attributed to the use of an essentially informal or unscientific approach.

The term 'assessment' is etymologically derived from the Latin *assidere* meaning to 'sit by' which denotes that some of its value relates to being supportively and empathically 'alongside' the person being assessed. Through this the client can, by the experience of being understood and accepted, be encouraged to develop a trusting therapeutic relationship with the nurse. However, it is no less likely that the nurse assessor and the wider service are also, ironically, being assessed as to their potential to understand, help and be trusted. The assessor is after all the representative of the service, being entrusted with the role of conducting the initial contact with the service in a manner that communicates competence.

Integral to the investigatory element of the assessment process is the quality of the information gleaned. It has to be sufficiently accurate and broad ranging for the nurse assessor to determine:

- whether there is a need for a nursing intervention
- the nature of the nursing intervention required.

Emphasizing the importance of the former is the increasing usage of the term 'treatment eligibility'. As a consequence a fiscal-conscious health service policy has dictated that mental health nurses, as with other occupational groups, move away from the notion of responding to all mental health-care needs to that of adopting stringent eligibility criteria. The assessment has to be sufficiently sophisticated to attribute a value to an individual's mental health status, thus indicating eligibility for services. Although for some reading this book, the stringent application of this is in sharp contrast to past or indeed recent clinical experience the belief in its necessity is by no means new. It was suggested nearly 30 years ago that eliciting the level of severity is an important element of assessment, offering the quasi-scientific equation of *severity = distress × uncontrollability × frequency* as a means to achieve this (Mehrabian 1970). Inherent in this shift in resource usage is of course the increased potential for the nursing intervention to be a non-response.

WHAT CONSTITUTES THE ASSESSMENT?

Having already established that assessment is a process based on investigation, what constitutes the assessment can be partly defined by the breadth of areas the nurse assessor seeks to investigate. Historically there has always been some disagreement within the various health-care professions as to the appropriate areas to assess and as such many students of whatever discipline do find it a complex and confusing area. Broadly speaking, however, the way in which people's health problems were traditionally viewed was for many years characterized by a polarizing nurture versus nature argument. This unfortunately often resulted in an ideologically biased assessment leading to the care not always being the most appropriate. However, as our understanding of the complexity of humanity has developed the shortcomings of this approach have become all too evident. In unison with this, nursing has met the challenge by adopting a holistic orientation.

Consequently, although this diversity and ineffability of the human condition will often mean the assessment task is a demanding one, it is important for the nurse assessor to maximize the unique and privileged opportunity that assessment affords by gleaning information that is multidimensional in its perspective. In other words, the nurse assessor should aim to elicit information that provides more than a superficial picture of the person's behaviour (as often seen in a medical diagnosis) by gaining a multidimensional understanding of the person's ability to perform self-care. One such multidimensional approach is the biological (sometimes seen as being analogous with physical), psychological and social (*biopsychosocial*) model. In essence, this takes the view that all human behaviour is driven by our biopsychosocial needs and as such our thoughts, feelings and behaviours are similarly influenced.

Inherent to this 'biopsychosocial' approach is the triadic relationship of its elements (Fig. 2.1). Although each element is potentially an influence in its own right, each can interact and so influence or be influenced by the others. Consequently, for the nurse assessor to only view the presence of the elements in isolation would be to potentially underplay their relevance and influence within the person's life. An obvious consequence of this shortfall would be an invalid nursing diagnosis and intervention.

NURSING DIAGNOSIS

It may be useful at this juncture to clarify the meaning of a nursing diagnosis. One way of looking at this is to consider one function of assessment as being to arrive at a conclusion or, as Barker (1997) has termed it, a judgement. However, possibly a more suitable way of describing this goal of assessment, one that uses existing medico-nursing terminology, is to call it a nursing diagnosis. To digress for a moment, some readers may see this idea of diagnosis, let alone judgement, as being at odds with the curative ethos of the nurse–patient relationship. Although it would be wrong and potentially dangerous to dismiss such arguments out of hand, the rejection of diagnosis and judgement as positive terms describing facets of assessment practice does unfortunately seem to be misguided, particularly when viewed as an ethical or philosophical issue. Arguably, in this instance, the problem is a semantic misunderstanding in which the terms are confused with 'being judgemental'.

Reinforcing this misunderstanding is the reality that these terms have become stereotyped as the preserve of the psychiatric medical profession. For nurses, this leads to a number of conceptual difficulties relating to elitism, paternalism and power (clearly the antithesis of the nurse–patient relationship). However, it also results in a clouding of the nurses' perception as to its use and value within assessment which can mask the fact, pointed out by Webb (1992), that in a number of significant ways the terms 'diagnosis' and 'problems' are interchangeable.

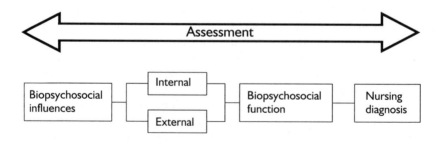

Figure 2.1 The biopsychosocial approach

However, as Savage (1991) notes, for nurses to use the term diagnosis authentically it is important to acknowledge that there are important features that separate the nursing diagnosis from the medical use of the term. The medical usage generally relies on categories based on symptom analysis. The nursing diagnosis, although not dismissive of the value of these, focuses on the person's response to their situation. In doing so it encourages the use of a far more descriptive language. In a sense the analogy of the difference between a newspaper headline and the body of its text holds true. The former, likened to the medical diagnosis, arguably provides only superficial stereotyped information with which to inform the reader as to whether the article is worth reading or not. Consequently, as it provides little height, length or breadth its limitations can result in it being as misinforming as it can be informing. In contrast, the nursing diagnosis describes reactions that link the cognitive, affective and behavioural response of the individual. In essence the nursing diagnosis is a statement that synthesizes the assessment information into a form that does not attempt to classify the person but conveys what Shannon *et al.* (1984) describe as the quality and context of the client's health and their responses to their circumstances. Defining this difference, Hogston (1997) highlights the incorporation of the phrase 'due to' within the nursing approach.

A BIOPSYCHOSOCIAL MODEL

Like any model, the biopsychosocial approach provides a framework within which information can be organized and categorized, thus making the information more manageable, easier to synthesize and so more meaningful (Fig 2.1). However, probably the most notable value to the assessment process that this particular approach offers is that it provides a framework that encompasses two equally determining components to a person's ability to self care: the biopsychosocial *influences* on the individual and the biopsychosocial *function* of the individual. Importantly, in the light of today's politicized climate, this second component is of significant value in determining current health status and, as such, eligibility. Nevertheless, both should be considered equally essential to the nurse assessor as both assist in developing an understanding of the contributing and maintaining factors to a person's problem(s), thus providing diagnostic reasoning to the intervention. It is, however, also important to consider the biopsychosocial influences as being twofold in their character: the internal and the external.

Internal influences

The internal element refers to those areas that are an integral part of the person's make-up, whether genetic or acquired. Biologically these can be considered to relate to the physical structure of the person and include such areas as the person's physical health (ill or otherwise), temporary or permanent disability, nutritional state, organic disorders, learning difficulties or disability, brain damage and sensory impairment (such as partial hearing or sight). Psychologically areas such as the person's intellectual capacity, personality, morality, values, nature of memories, integration of past experiences, self-identity, self-assigned roles and emotional make-up are all areas that can be considered internal influences.

External influences

External biological factors include the influence of the physical environment on self-care, e.g., access to warmth and shelter, past events/traumas, how others interact with the individual, how societal values define role and status. Socially the individual's network of human relationships (family or otherwise), their integration or acceptance within this network and their assigned roles all contribute to the ability to perform self-care.

Biopsychosocial function

Functionally the biopsychosocial approach assists the nurse assessor to understand the impact of the influences on the individual. Areas such as those highlighted below are of value in determining the individual's adaptation to internal and external influences. Those areas the nurse assessor should consider when using a biopsychosocial approach to assessment include the following.

Biological
- *Sleep* – duration, quality of, presence and type of insomnia (e.g. initial, middle, late), significant dreams
- *Diet* – interest, intake, weight loss/gain, potential influences on health, e.g. quality of diet, caffeine intake
- *Drug use* – (prescribed, illicit, alcohol, nicotine)
- *Physical health* – significant illnesses, general level of health
- *Physical symptoms* (somatic) – panic attacks/anxiety (duration, frequency, intensity, occurrence), headaches

Psychological
- *Speech* – form, flow and content
- Any impairment of *concentration, memory*
- *Self-perception* – sense of identity, spirituality (secular or religious)
- *Motivation, attitude*
- *Mood*:
    Cognition – suicidal ideation, homicidal ideation, thought disorder, self-perception, perceived perception of self by others
    Anhedonia
    Hallucinations
    Diurnal variation in mood
- *Behaviour*:
    Non-verbal communication
    Speech – form/flow/content
    Avoidances, excesses

Social

- *Significant relationships* – nature and quality of family, social, work, forensic history
- *Occupational/time structuring* – nature and value
- *Financial situation*
- *Housing/environment* – nature and quality of relationship

THE ART AND SCIENCE OF ASSESSMENT

How are needs identified? What helps the nurse assessor decide when a client's presenting issue merits service intervention? Within psychiatric mental health nursing, where the nurse is in a position of significant influence, the traditional responses to these questions have been frequently heavily weighted towards subjectivity and the nurse's perception. However, within a climate of resource limitations and the need for reliability and validity, subjectivity could be regarded as at best a useful but limited adjunct but at worst a dangerously misguiding tool. So in order to ensure its usefulness is maximized it is important that it partners a methodology that is at least partly based on scientific reasoning.

The reader may at this point be asking themselves whether an emphasis on a systematic approach could be overformal and the simple answer is yes it most certainly can if approached from a purist's perspective. Therefore, in order to avoid this, it is essential for the nurse assessor to remember that one of the purposes of the assessment is to establish a therapeutic relationship with the client. For this to happen successfully requires a component that is not usually considered a natural bedfellow of a formal or scientific methodology – the human touch.

Although this element is often regarded as the therapeutic use of appropriate eye contact, a smile, a nod or an empathic response, there is another dimension to it that is equally valuable to the role – the use of the intuition skills of the nurse assessor. To explain further, the formal approach in one sense can be considered analogous to a scientific approach – a systematic and formulated enquiry, whereas intuition or 'understanding without reasoning' can be considered as being akin to the art of nursing – the human component.

Interestingly, many nurses do in fact consider their practice to be primarily intuition led (Appleton 1993). However, although authors such as Morse *et al.* (1994) have suggested that nurses often have the ability to state the patient's condition without the symptoms being explicitly reported, the nurse assessor should be aware of the limitations and pitfalls of relying on intuition if they are to successfully harness its true value. With this in mind the nurse assessor should harness both a technical rationality (scientific approach) as described by Kelly (1997) whilst developing, with an awareness of the weighting given to it within their own practice, an intuitive or informal approach.

It is, however, important to note that the objectivity that is offered by the scientific approach is also not infallible and can be similarly prone to the bias and prejudice sometimes attributed to the unreasoned knowledge provided through intuition. For example, the personalized way of using investigatory tools can result in a significant variability. Similarly, the nuances inherent in the client's presentation of themselves can often only be picked up through the use of human touch.

Therefore, although it would be folly to omit intuition from any form of interpersonal relationship in which understanding and empathy are of paramount importance, its value and its use should be reflective of its limited objectivity, validity and uncertain reliability. However, as a word of caution, it is important to note that the information collection function of assessment should, as Savage (1991) suggests, be objectified rather than a purely objective process. If this is achieved the assessment and by association mental health nursing as a process can move closer to what Barker and Johnson (1996) term as the most scientific of the humanities and the most humane of the sciences and thus 'come of age'.

CONDUCTING AN ASSESSMENT

The assessment should routinely cover additional areas such as demographic details, reason for referral (the referrer may have a specific objective in mind), the client's understanding of the problem and when the problem began. Additionally the nurse assessor should glean an understanding of what the client has already tried in order to resolve or cope with the problem.

Depending on the area in which the assessment is taking place, information may already have been collected by other professionals. The Nurse Assessor should therefore be prepared to obtain this information prior to assessment, clarify its accuracy and include it in the assessment report where appropriate. It may also be useful to involve family, carers and/or friends in the assessment if agreed upon with the client. However, if the assessed is, due to their mental state, considered to be either at or potentially at serious risk, possibly because they are not in touch with reality, it may be appropriate for the nurse assessor to act in 'good faith' and in enacting their duty of care obtain necessary information from others even without the client's knowledge or consent. This area is understandably fraught with moral, ethical and legal issues and it may be appropriate to discuss this with the nursing or multidisciplinary team prior to obtaining such information.

Any information collected is of course of limited value if it is less than accurate or incomplete. An essential ingredient in avoiding, or at least minimizing, such an outcome is through the nurse assessor quickly establishing a therapeutic alliance with the client so that the client feels accepted, understood and above all safe. Undoubtedly the main tool at the disposal of the nurse assessor is the focused and therapeutic use of interpersonal skills.

Methods of collecting assessment information

As already stated, a primary function of assessment is to learn about the client through investigation which requires the collection of accurate and relevant information. However, in order to achieve this the assessment methodology has to be appropriate not only to the assessment's purpose but also to the environment in which it is to be used, e.g. community clinic, client's home, ward or residential setting. All of these will have common characteristics but they will also provide their own peculiarities and idiosyncrasies. For example, in some instances the nurse assessor may gain additional information through the presence of relatives, carers or friends (this can be of great value when the client's mental state may restrict their ability to communicate). Another setting may provide important information relating to the influence of the environment on the situation. The ability of the nurse assessor to be sensitive and receptive of this will have a bearing on the flow and effectiveness of the assessment.

Although the framework employed by the nurse assessor needs to be planned (as opposed to *ad hoc*) it should also be appropriate and sufficiently adaptable to the needs and abilities of the client. The nurse assessor needs to have the capacity to reflect in practice (Schon 1983); that is, to have on-the-spot awareness in order to appropriately adjust to the client and their environment as necessary. An example would be the necessity for the nurse assessor to take account of impaired cognitive function, as is common in depression or psychosis, or the client's emotional state, both of which may impair their ability to 'tell their story'. In short, the assessment should not be conducted in a rigid, robotic or regimented way, merely presented as a list of closed questions.

However, at the other end of the competent assessment/poor assessment continuum, the absence of a systemized assessment model could be likened to hurriedly attempting to complete a complex jigsaw puzzle. When embarking on such a task it can be tempting to quickly scan all the pieces in order to try and mentally construct the finished picture. When this proves unsuccessful it can be further tempting for the puzzler (the assessor) to attempt, again mentally, to categorize the pieces in the hope of finding a short route to determining the completed image (diagnosis). However, unless the nurse is blessed with enormous luck, these processes tend only to provide at best partial success and at worst an abstract and confused picture (misdiagnosis). Therefore, in order to achieve the desired outcome (an accurate diagnosis), the puzzler is usually forced to backtrack and adopt a methodological approach that is essentially systematic.

Similarly this *ad hoc* or informal approach has the potential to result in the information gleaned being misunderstood. As with the sightseer in Stevie Smith's evocative poem 'Not waving but drowning', the view of a swimmer from what seems a good vantage point on the cliff top seems clear. However, unable to pick out important details, the bystander interprets the arm gesticulations incorrectly, thus tragically misunderstanding the communication and therefore the situation. Needless to say, misunderstanding the client's information in a similar way can also have tragic consequences.

So, in order to avoid the pitfalls that such an approach encourages, the nurse assessor attempting to investigate and understand accurately the client and their problems requires an approach that is scientific and systematic. One such approach is the triangulated methodology advocated by Savage (1991) and Milne (1993). Unsurprisingly, this approach, incorporating observation, a semi-structured interview and the use of rating scales or inventories, is generally considered far more likely to yield reliable and valid information than an *ad hoc* assessment and, as with the puzzler's plight, it is also probably the least frustrating method of investigation and collection. In order for this approach to be truly beneficial it requires familiarity with the process and practice. The nurse assessor should therefore not be put off by the potential for not recalling the breadth of information required in order for the assessment to be considered holistic.

Rating scales

The value of including validated rating scales or questionnaires is essentially twofold. First, their use provides a tool by which the nurse assessor can elicit information about a client's health status in a standardized format. This not only helps focus the assessment onto measurable areas but also provides information that can be used at a later date to evaluate the effectiveness of treatment. The former also has the potential to be a catalyst for further or deeper enquiry into the client's difficulties. Second, although the information collected is a subjective measurement of the client's reality (Barker 1997) it is nevertheless the client's perspective of their symptoms or situation and as such establishes a starting point for treatment. Although this subjectivity is often cited as a reason not to use rating scales, it is important to remember that no assessment can be devoid of subjectivity. To adapt Winston Churchill's adage on democracy, there is no such thing as a non-subjective assessment, there are only some that are less subjective than others.

Although many nurses are thought to be prejudiced against rating scales and questionnaires, believing that they block the development of the nurse–client relationship, the contrary is often true. In rating scales such as the Hospital Anxiety and Depression Scale (HAD) or the Beck Depression Inventory (BDI), the mere fact that the client sees their symptoms in print often elicits a response similar to that observed in supportive group work when the universalities of human experience are acknowledged through sharing. The resultant internal 'sigh of relief' that says 'I'm not alone in having these feelings' can be considered as a therapeutic milestone, one that helps develop a sense of being understood. This undoubtedly assists the establishment of the therapeutic relationship and the success of any subsequent treatment.

Rating scales in the form of record sheets or diaries can also be utilized as a means of self-monitoring or of helping the client achieve goals. Probably the most obvious application of these is in a systematic desensitization programme in which the client is asked to record their progress on a daily basis. In this instance the feedback provided by the recorded information is an encouragement to develop a positive internal dialogue. If the client does not achieve their goals, this can be used with the nurse to identify problem areas.

Observation

This is probably the most universally employed form of intervention within a nursing assessment and is probably also the oldest. However, although it relies on what is often wrongly considered to be something everyone does competently without any training, i.e. use of one's eyes and ears, its value within assessment remains unique. It occurs before the formality of the assessment has begun (e.g. how the person walks into the room, how they respond to your greeting or for that matter how they greet you) and carries on throughout the assessment.

For observation to be effective, the nurse assessor must be aware of the subtleties of non-verbal communication, e.g. the anxious client wringing their hands when talking about a particular subject, and visual information such as clothing, rings that no longer fit through weight loss, dark rings around the eyes or predominantly thoracic breathing.

Assessment tools

Reliability

A reliable tool provides consistent results on repeated administration, i.e. if the same client were to use the tool a number of times any variation in the results would be minimal. Milne (1993) illustrates the importance of this using the analogy of taking measurements using an elastic band. By the very nature of the elastic band's construction there is a high probability that the user will not be provided with information that can be comparable. In effect, as a measuring tool it is unreliable.

Validity

This is essentially whether the tool measures what it claims to measure. For example, does it actually measure levels of depression or does it allow unwanted, unnecessary or distorting information to contaminate the results? An aspect of this could be the potential for human bias in interpretation of the findings. Significant bias would render the information invalid.

Although there are many assessment tools available, the simpler the tool, the easier it will be incorporate it into the assessment interview. This also allows it to be used in such a way that it does not take over the assessment and so undermine the interpersonal component of the assessment. The following tools are representative of those currently available.

Hamilton Depression Scale (HDS)

This is an assessor-rated scale and as such is not particularly easy to incorporate into the face-to-face component of the assessment. It is primarily designed to be used as a means of quantifying the results of the assessment and relies heavily on the skill of the assessor to elicit during the assessment the necessary information covered in the scale.

Beck Depression Inventory (BDI)

This is possibly one of the best known rating scales. In its original form it comprised 21 questions designed to assess the severity of depression through cognition and mood. It includes items about mood, sleep and self-perception. A more recent user-friendly version of 12 items is now more commonly employed.

Both are scored by summing up the ratings on a four-point scale ranging from 0–3. Answers are based on how the person has felt over the previous week. The shortened version has a maximum score of 21. Scores from 0–4 are considered within the normal range or asymptomatic, scores of 5–7 indicate mild depression while scores of 8–15 indicate moderate depression; scores of 16 or more indicate severe depression.

Hospital Anxiety Depression Scale (HADS)

As with the BDI, this is a self-report questionnaire designed to be a detection tool. Again, as with the BDI, it uses how the person has felt over the previous week in order to screen for symptoms. Although titled as a hospital scale it lends itself well to the community setting. Its 14 questions equally identify levels of anxiety and depression, focusing on attitude and somatic symptoms. Each question has three options to choose from which identify behaviours and mood. Final scoring utilizes three bands that indicate the probability of no anxiety or depression being present (0–7), a borderline presence (8–11) or a significant presence (12–21).

General Health Questionnaire (GHQ)

Generally considered as being the most effective screening tool, its main use is in a primary care setting. Being essentially a screening tool for use with the general population, its questions are very broad ranging. The questionnaire provides the assessor with subtotals on four scales and an overall total score. A somatic scale contains questions about the person's feelings providing a measure of the bodily sensations that usually occur at times of emotional upset. The anxiety scale focuses on anxiety and sleeplessness whereas the social scale measures the impact on usual challenges of life. The fourth scale measures depression and encompasses suicidal ideation. The total score measures the probability measure of psychiatric 'caseness'. Although considered to have good reliability and validity, its original 60-item questionnaire has proved difficult to integrate into both general and specialist assessments. As with the BDI, a shorter version comprising 28 questions has been developed.

Edinburgh Postnatal Depression Scale (EPDS)

The EPDS is a simple and straightforward questionnaire designed to be completed in a relatively short time. Studies have shown it to be as effective a screening tool, in terms of reliability and validity, as many of the more established tools.

Social Adaptation Self-evaluation Scale (SASS)

This is considered to be a relatively user-friendly rating scale designed to measure social functioning as an outcome measure in depression. It consists of 21 simple questions which, unlike most other questionnaires, are not symptom orientated. It explores the four main areas of social functioning, i.e. work, leisure time, family and coping ability with resources and finance. Questions relating to these headings are not clustered in order to ensure questions are answered independently. Each item scores 0–3; the higher the score, the better the level of functioning. Normal social functioning range is considered to lie between 35 and 52 out of a possible 63.

Interviewing and communication skills

First impressions count or so it is said. Indeed, it is suggested here that the proficiency in conducting an assessment is often contingent upon how one starts it off. By now, it should be clear what the authors' position is as regards assessment: namely, that assessment provides a positive foundation for relationship building and, conversely, the establishment of rapport is a necessary springboard for competent assessment. How, then, to go about establishing rapport, that indefinable quality so beloved of counselling textbooks? One way, of course, is to 'skirt around' the issue in what Burnard (1991) refers to as 'pussyfooting' or at least to resort to small-talk on everything but the person's problem. The principle involved is that of 'warming up' the interviewee by talking on 'safe' matters, such as the weather or the journey taken to see you (unless you've gone to the client), with a view to gradually developing directness. The difficulty here is the obfuscation that may result, neither interviewer or interviewee being clear about the purpose of the interview. This gives rise to what Barker (1997, p. 20) refers to as 'Kipling's six honest serving men', i.e. six questions vital to assessment, which are: what, why, when, how, where and who? The second of these is the concern here: why? Or, more specifically, why am I doing this assessment? This question acts as a built-in check. If the assessor's answer is, 'I don't know', something has gone seriously wrong!

This is not justification for swinging towards the other extreme, usually referred to as the 'sledgehammer' approach. Assessment is not interrogation and a propensity for 'leading' questions can do untold damage. A 'too much too soon' style of assessment such as this can result in anything but rapport, when frustration at unmet expectations could give rise to a marked degree of tension, which could so easily have been avoided. This possibility is particularly pertinent in the context of community mental health-care politics, in which attention is focused upon the most severe problem of the individual, specifically in terms of risk and potential threat to public safety. It becomes apparent that all the 'actors' in the assessment process need to be clear, as far as possible, about what is happening and what the purpose of assessment is in relation to the care process in general. By such means, in ideal circumstances at least, a mutual understanding of the basic principles of assessment can be gained and other benefits, which are byproducts of the process and yet are crucial, such as consent, collaboration and consensus, can be facilitated. It now is necessary to indicate how all this can be achieved, with the intention of finding a way through the impasse created by the two extremes of 'pussyfooting' in contrast to the interrogative 'sledgehammer' style.

'How can I help you?' is an example of how we can learn from the techniques of the service industries. It is an open question and thus acts as a lever for an extensive response. The drawback is, of course, that it lends itself to the shortcut, plunging straight into planning and implementing care before a thorough assessment has taken place. It's worth repeating once again that skilled implementation of care is contingent upon skilled assessment. 'What has brought you along to see me?' is a useful open-ended way of starting off the interview and has the advantage of being geared to the assessment as such, rather than care planning. On the other hand, it has little value with people who, to a minor extent, do not acknowledge their need for help and in the extreme, actively resist any offers of help. Nevertheless, such a way of starting the interview does underwrite the individualized nature of assessment and provides a platform for the holistic movement, serving as an antithesis of the medical model, noted for its impersonal approach in the rush towards classification. Holism is necessarily related to individualism. It is the disparate parts that go towards forming the person and yet, interestingly, the individual is something more than the person. In such a way, individualized care produces, and is reproduced by, the uniqueness of the individual.

'Tell me about yourself' is invariably a sound start to the assessment interview, in that it eschews preconceived ideas. Yet another advantage of this particular 'lead-in' is its avoidance of what the behaviourists call deficits and medical personnel call symptoms. It is driven by the tenet of the 'patient' as a person. It would be unfortunate were mental health nurses to forego this 'opener' in assessment in the name of economy. It is imperative not to lose sight of the person in the mounting pressure to assess primarily in terms of risk. As a criticism, this question may be too broad and steer the interviewee away from the intended focus towards largely irrelevant 'tributaries' of data.

It is as well to argue now that assessment of every last detail of one person is both unsustainable and, frankly, unwise. Thus an ideal opportunity is provided at this point to discuss questioning technique and how it is irrevocably linked with listening.

Questioning technique

Skilled questioning is only as good as the listening that accompanies it. The wisdom of being brief and explicit in one's questioning is related to the likelihood of clients being reticent in answering questions, through embarrassment, low self-esteem, an expectation of not being understood or the likelihood of stigmatization. Clients as disempowered people not only lack a voice but in time begin to internalize that they are not deserving of one. As Freire (1962) reminds us, it is only through education that the oppressed, and clients are widely held to be in this category (Faulkner and Sayce 1997), can begin to be empowered. The multiple or long rambling question will only serve to obfuscate the intended meaning; this does nothing to put the service user at ease. Indeed, the result may be quite the reverse and the interviewee might well become suspicious or retreat into silence. This doesn't mean, of course, that probing questions of the 'Did you have sex last night?' kind are in order. They are, almost always, not acceptable!

This is where we come to the open question, long regarded as the most fruitful, in terms of gathering information. It is worthwhile at this point illustrating what the open question has to offer. Open questions have two distinct advantages. First, the questioner is likely to be perceived as human and, by implication, approachable. As Barker (1997) suggests, such qualities are currently placed in some opposition to the competency of the 'psychotechnician', who is much more likely to concentrate on closed, specific questions. The client is going to feel understood when asked an open question, as it is much more conducive to active listening. In fact, the two actions, asking open questions and active listening, are closely intertwined.

Second, open questions enable the interviewee to gain some control and thus become more self-determined. This is where we can learn from field research methods of investigation. Burgess (1984) points to the unstructured interview in terms of 'the interview as conversation'. A great deal of listening is implicated here. In this section it has been argued that this 'facilitative' style is essential in building trust within the early development of the therapeutic relationship, within which the assessment process is central. The effective listener is found by people in crisis to be more supportive (Truax and Carkhuff 1967). One qualification, however: open questioning is not meant to be synonymous with multiple or long-winded questioning. It must be focused and yet not probing.

In summary, the open style of questioning creates more comfort and is conducive to a collaborative partnership. This means that controversies rage within mental health nursing in general, and assessment in particular, as to whether formal methods of assessments are the way forward or whether the traditional reverence of informal assessment needs to be upheld. Mental health nurses, with growing experience and confidence, frequently therefore adapt their style of assessment and the communication skills used during the assessment process to suit the needs of the client and the context in which the assessment takes place.

REFERENCES

Appleton, C. (1993) The art of nursing: the experience of patients and nurses. *Journal of Advanced Nursing* 18: 892–899.

Barker, P. (1997) *The Assessment Process in Mental Health Nursing*. Stanley Thornes, Cheltenham.

Barker, P. and Johnson, T. (1996) Seriously misguided. *Nursing Times* 92(34): 56–57.

Burgess, R. (1984) *In the Field*. Allen and Unwin, London.

Burnard, P. (1991) *Caring and Communicating*. Macmillan, Basingstoke.

Burns, T. (1994) Mrs Bottomley's ten point plan. *Psychiatric Bulletin* 18: 129–130.

Burns, T. (1997) Case management, care management and care programming. *British Journal of Psychiatry* 170: 393–395.

Dobson, F. (1998) *Strategy Launched to Modernise Mental Health Services*. Department of Health, London.

DoH (1990) *The Care Programme Approach for People with a Mental Illness Referred to the Specialist Services*. HC(90)23/LASSL(90). HMSO, London.

DoH (1991) *Access to Health Records Act – A Guide for the NHS*. Department of Health, London.

DoH (1994) *Mental Illness Key Areas Handbook*. HMSO, London.

DoH (1995) *Building Bridges – The Health of the Nation*. Department of Health, London.

Faulkner, A. and Sayce, L. (1997) Disclosure. *Open Mind* **85**: 8–9.

Freire, P. (1962) *The Pedagogy of the Oppressed*. Penguin, Harmondsworth.

Hogston, R. (1997) Nursing diagnosis and classification systems: a positional paper. *Journal of Advanced Nursing* **26**: 496–500.

Huxley, P. (1990) Community mental health: a challenge to care. *Community Psychiatric Nursing Journal* **10**(3): 61–63.

Kelly, A. (1997) The concept of the specialist community nurse. *Journal of Advanced Nursing* **24**: 42–52.

Lingham, R., Candy, J. and Bray, J. (1996) *Report of the Inquiry into the Treatment and Care of Raymond Sinclair*. West Kent Health Authority and Kent County Council, Maidstone.

Mehrabian, B. (1970) *Tactics of Social Influence*. Prentice Hall, New Jersey.

Milne, D. (1993) *Psychology and Mental Health Nursing*. Macmillan, London.

Moore, C. and Wolf, J. (1999) Open and shut case. *Health Service Journal* **24 June**: 108–110.

Morrall, P. (1995) Clinical autonomy and the community psychiatric nurse. *mental Health Nursing*, **15**(2): 16–19.

Morse, J., Miles, W., Cark, A. and Doberneck, B. (1994) Sensing patient needs: exploring concepts of nursing insight and receptivity used in nursing assessment. *Scholarly Inquiry for Nursing Practice: An International Journal* **8**(3): 233–253.

Onyett, S. (1992) *Case Management in Mental Health*. Chapman and Hall, London.

Ritchie, J.H., Dick, D. and Lingham, R. (1994) *Report of the Inquiry into the Care and Treatment of Christopher Clunis*. HMSO, London.

Rose, N. (1986) Law, rights and psychiatry. In: Miller, P. and Rose, N. (eds) *The Power of Psychiatry*. Polity Press, Cambridge.

Savage, P. (1991) Patient assessment in psychiatric nursing. *Journal of Advanced Nursing* **16**: 311–316.

Schon, D. (1983) *The Reflective Practitioner*. Basic Books, New York.

Shannon, C., Wahl, P., Rhea, M. and Dyehouse, J. (1984) The nursing process. In: Beck, C. et al. (eds) *Mental Health Psychiatric Nursing*. Mosby, St Louis.

Stein, L.I. and Test, M.A. (19890) Alternatives to mental hospital treatment. I Conceptual model, treatment programme and clinical evaluation. *Archives of General Psychiatry* **37**: 392–397.

Truax, C.B. and Carkhuff, R.R. (1967) *Towards Effective Counselling and Psychotherapy*. Aldine Press, Chicago.

Webb, C. (1992) … or two steps back? *Nursing Times* **7**(88): 33–34.

3 THE NURSE AS EDUCATOR

Richard Barrett

OBJECTIVES

After reading this chapter, you should be able to:

- identify the role of the clinician in the education of students and health workers in outcome-based assessment of practice
- critically examine the position of the nurse as a trainer of practice in the current shift towards practice-based education
- discuss the value of recent professional developments in mental health care and their impact on the nurse's role as mentor
- evaluate the mental health nurse's significance as a role model in light of the emergence of the supervision model in nurse education
- identify how the nurse's role in therapeutic interventions is a feature in client education
- discuss the potential of the mental health nurse in the field of health promotion.

INTRODUCTION

In the expected transition to a more practice-based preregistration education (ENB 2000) the mental health nurse as educator has a key role. The nurse as educator involves two basic elements: that of instructor, imparting skills and knowledge to those less experienced, situated anywhere on the continuum from novice to expert (Benner 1984) and that of health promoter, seeking to foster the promotion of mental health and the prevention of mental illness. This chapter will embrace both elements of the educator role. The full remit of this role is very extensive, so an attempt will be made to separate the nurse as instructor from the nurse as health promoter, even though this is a false dichotomy given the overlap between the two elements. There is also a tension between calls for curricula to be health based (ENB 2000, UKCC 1986) and recommendations for mental health nurses to focus on the care of the severely mentally ill (DoH 1998b). Proposals for change must not compromise the need for an ever more informed general public in terms of mental *health*. In this context, *The Health of the Nation* (DoH 1994a) and, more recently, *Our Healthier Nation* (DoH 1998a) underline that the development of the mental health nurse's role as educator is long overdue, hence the emphasis on health promotion in Standard One of the National Service Framework's first national standards for mental health (DoH 1999b).

The first section of this chapter will look at the nurse's role as trainer, exploring the challenges of a learning domain in which the emergence of the health worker is paramount (Sainsbury Centre for Mental Health 1997, DoH 2000). It is expected that in future, the nurse as educator, in common with the other aspects of being a nurse, will be located in a multiprofessional and multiagency network (DoH 1996). Following this section, the nurse as role model will be critically evaluated. Will the nurse's skills be eroded further? Or, on the contrary, does the nurse have current, appropriate and observable skills through which others can learn? The focus then switches to identifying how the nurse as therapist can be an educator, first through giving advice and information in groups and secondly through family-based interventions. In the background is a paradox between expectations of the professionalization of nurses and greater service user involvement in policies and provision of care, and the impact of this paradox on practice-based care (UKCC 1999) will need to be considered. The recommendations for closer links between the primary care and secondary care sectors will also need to be brought into the equation.

The remainder of the chapter will explore the nurse as educator in terms of health promotion. It is intended to utilize Caplan's (1964) model of preventive psychiatry for a host of reasons, not least because it is relevant to the way mental health care is delivered, despite being overlooked by government recommendations for changes in health-care policy. Caplan enables the incorporation of health promotion into the primary level of prevention by way of others' (Tudor 1996) development of the theory. Fundamentally, Caplan provides a framework, involving secondary and tertiary levels, which can be analysed in light of current and proposed shifts in care delivery towards greater collaboration. This shift to a more democratic, less hierarchical care structure has as its bedrock the nurse, who occupies a pivotal position in the matrix of diverse interest groups. The nurse's position as trainer represents a particular example of this pivotal role and will now be considered.

THE TRAINER

Since its move into higher education institutions (HEIs) following the advent of Project 2000 (UKCC 1986) nurse education has become increasingly academic, so much so that concerns have been raised around the level of practice skills of nurses achieving registration (DoH 1999a, ENB 2000, UKCC 1999). Yet even with a greater emphasis on theory, the concept of training persists, given that nursing continues to be conceptualized at one extreme as fundamentally a practical activity (Sharp 1995) and more accurately as a synthesis of theory *and* practice. Equally, the development of practice skills requires training, as distinct from education. The trainer is defined as: 'One who trains; esp. one who prepares men, horses, etc., for races etc.' (*The Concise English Dictionary* 1994). The implication is that the trainer gives instruction, in contrast to the educator, who may incorporate the role of trainer but has, in addition, a responsibility for the intellectual and moral development of those being educated. Put another way, a trainer imparts 'how to do' something whereas the educator explains the principles underlying that which is to be performed, in facilitating students' development of critical thinking.

This section will explore the move to professionalization of mental health nurses and its link with the training process. A complex matrix of theoretical and philosophical perspectives has developed, such that training will be influenced by, but not necessarily overwhelmed with, any one single value position; the nurse will be informed by a range of contested positions, each claiming access to 'the truth'. Nursing has long given rise to, and been shaped by, a pluralistic philosophical framework (Barker 1990) and there is every reason to believe that the nurse will continue to confront a multiplicity of perspectives, given the range of educational innovations that have emerged in the last 30 years or so. Just one example is the humanistic perspective, which was initially very influential in counselling, giving rise to the person-centred approach (Rogers 1967) and more recently in relation to education, in which student-centredness has become a key feature (Rogers 1983).

Not only are training principles worthy of consideration in this section but also the learning environment in which training takes place will require examination in regard particularly to who might be the key player in training. Finally, the emphasis being placed on multidisciplinary training in a succession of recommendations for the development of mental health care will require analysis, if only because such changes will inevitably impact on the training of nurses.

Training, in the sense of instructing junior staff on their practical performance, as defined above, is increasingly assessment-driven. Moreover, practice assessment itself is monopolized largely by behavioural outcomes (Milligan 1998) which seek to assess *performance* rather than skills as such. This highlights a dichotomy for the trainer between solely work-related skills (practice) and theory. Milligan (1998) argues that this is a false dichotomy which has been perpetuated in nurse education for too long. Thinking on this has long overlooked a working model which adequately integrates the two elements in assessment, i.e. theory and practice. *Competency* is a term commonly used to suggest an integration of practice with theory and indeed Schon (1983) alone indicates that competency is constituted of various forms of knowledge which underlie the successful and adaptive performance of skills (Milligan 1998). Current proposals for the reform of preregistration nurse education do not emphasize the place of theory in the development of competence. The newly qualified nurse is seen to be competent if possessing 'the skills and ability to practise safely and efficiently without the need for direct supervision' (UKCC 1999).

NVQ training presents a case in point. Confusion is evident in the sphere of training for mental health care, in that the assessment of *competencies* is seen as central to the process. Yet at the same time, successful performance rests only on *being able to do it* with no regard for the independence of mind or critical thinking implied by a knowledge base. This has relevance to the nurse as trainer in terms of the whole issue of professionalization, if only for the fact that NVQ training serves as a boundary between professional and non-professional, regardless of greater democratization within the mental health-care network. Freidson (1972) emphasizes this distinction when he points to a specialized body of knowledge as a characteristic of a profession. Again, the nurse is positioned as a key player in training, yet is often concerned to develop academically, with more and more emphasis on ever higher levels of qualifications. However, in the practice setting the clinician has tremendous leverage in determining the extent to which nurses become empowered and, as indicated later in this section, is pivotal in the development of mental health care now and in the future.

Increasingly, the nurse trainer is expected to adopt the principle of mentorship, which is to do with guiding, in addition to assessing the outcomes of the individual. By so doing, the nurse should take heed of the shift towards adult education (Knowles 1990), involving the principle of androgogy, which sees the trainee as a central figure in his or her assessment. In this way, the self-assessment of the health-care worker/student nurse/newly qualified nurse serves as a parallel to the care process itself, in which the client takes an active part in the planning and implementation of his own care and in the broader picture may choose to be involved in the development of mental health-care policy as a whole.

It is important to remember that assessment must involve an ongoing dialogue between trainer and trainee. It is designed to address any concerns about performance earlier rather than later. The ongoing nature of practice assessment is significant and such significance must be recognized so as to understand it as a positive, developmental process. If this advice is followed the trainer will adopt a problem-solving strategy, being able to negotiate with the trainee so that a consensus can be achieved. Thus the horrors of past practice assessment (in the pre-mentorship era), which could involve overly negative and, above all, belated feedback to the trainee, should not occur in the contemporary context of assessment which rests on partnership, not pedagogy.

This representation of the training dyad, in which both parties participate actively, parallels the nurse–client relationship but is differentiated by the fact that the trainee has a responsibility to be evaluated. The client, in contrast, is assessed but not evaluated. Responsibility of the trainee involves insight into his or her strengths and weaknesses, representing an integral part of self-directed learning.

None of the above should divert us from the context in which the nurse as trainer is located; it is important at this point to give consideration to the political and economic factors which impact on the learning environment and the context in which such learning takes place, essentially a professionalized one. In common with other professions, and indeed in its attempt to emulate them, nursing has of late adopted many of their features. It is essential to view such developments as advances in mental health nursing which at one stage could only have been dreamt about. In particular, *The Code of Professional Conduct* (UKCC 1992) is underpinned by the maxim that autonomy cannot exist without accountability. Cooperation with colleagues in what is essentially a team activity is enshrined within this document. Equally, the nurse has an ethical and legal responsibility to develop the future lifeblood of the profession of nursing, given the shortfall of nurses registering with the UKCC between 1993–94 and 1997–98 (UKCC 1999). Teaching and assessing has become an integral part of the clinician's role. The ENB 1998 course 'Teaching and Learning in Clinical Practice' has become a central feature of role development but a fundamental shift in policy is evident in Recommendation 28 of *Fitness for Practice* (UKCC 1999) which proposes that preparation, support of and feedback to mentors by lecturers needs to be formalized and continued in preceptorship.

It should be apparent in the discussion so far that the trainer's role extends far beyond the capacity of assessor. Notable developments that inveigh against mere assessment of the trainee's capacity to perform learning outcomes and more towards a mentoring role are the incorporation of clinical supervision (Rolfe 1990, Severinsson 1998), reflective practice (Haddock 1997) and preceptorship into the training realm. These must now be considered in turn, before illustrating how such development is not linear in nature and is subject to a conflict of interests. Other specific developments will be cited as a way of illustrating how mental health nurses are gaining much enhanced recognition in the health-care domain.

Preregistration nurse education is open to criticism by being overly concerned with assessment, causing the student nurse to focus solely on achieving learning outcomes at the expense of other modes of learning. Proposals to make preregistration education more outcome-based (ENB 2000) are expected to give assessment an even higher profile. Learning outcomes are not individualized and lead to a degree of uniformity, even when achieved in different settings. Moreover, assessment schedules imply that all students understand, progress towards and achieve outcomes at the same time, which is clearly not the case. Individuals very markedly in the pace at which they learn. The bureaucratization of learning points to a standardization of learning characterized by fixed criteria. On the other hand, recommendations for flexibility in entry to preregistration education does acknowledge students' different speeds of learning and prior experience. Clinical supervision has a distinct advantage in that it is individualized and, above all, is not assessment driven.

In order to be an effective supervisor, one must first of all establish a climate of trust. This is easier said than done yet is an aspect that is often overlooked. Severinsson (1998), for example, focuses so much on procedural aspects of group supervision in her study of supervision of Swedish student nurses (across a wide range of care settings) that she overlooks the interpersonal process completely. All the more surprisingly, Severinsson advocates a pedagogic approach. This is unlikely to make trainees feel at ease. It is becoming increasingly essential to adopt an adult education format (Knowles 1990) and as Rogers (1983) has found, people learn best when they have control over and choice in what they learn. Equally, the person-centred model of clinical supervision (Dexter and Wash 1995) posits the core conditions (Rogers 1967) – genuineness, empathy and unconditional positive regard – as fundamental to the teacher's facilitation of student-centredness in clinical supervision. On the whole, trainees do not readily bring problems to supervision of their own initiative; they often need some help to do so!

It is possible that a pedantic approach to supervision is equated with professional status. This is quite erroneous, illustrated by the fact that much of the professional cachet of mental health nurses is their capacity to be everything other than pedagogic. On the other hand, if the safety of the client/s and others is being jeopardized, it is justifiable, indeed it is the duty of the supervisor to acknowledge and respond to concerns being brought to supervision by the supervisee, essentially within the realms of confidentiality. Power (1999, p. 124) advises that the agreement of confidentiality should only be broken when the supervisor considers that the supervisee has disclosed or demonstrated professional misconduct and/or that he is unfit to practise nursing for reasons of ill health. The 'duty to care', indirect or otherwise, is paramount. The nurse is no less accountable as a supervisor having a responsibility to give positive advice in such instances, in light of having greater experience and knowledge than the supervisee (Wright *et al.* 1997). Specified *consistent* clinical supervision is a central feature of the transition towards practice-based education (ENB 2000).

Who is best positioned to undertake such training strategies as highlighted above? Clinicians who are authorized mentors are ideally placed to undertake such initiatives. First, they are in direct contact with clients, unlike nurse lecturers. Many lecturers have abdicated the traditional role of clinical teachers, coinciding, it would seem, with the amalgamation of nurse training into higher education, so much so that a major strand of proposals for nurse education (UKCC 1999) recommends a greater involvement of lecturers in practice. This is to be achieved through close consultation between service providers and health education institutions. A parallel development has seen the appointment of educational facilitators in service provision. In centres of learning the appointment of lecturer practitioners is advised (DoH 1999a) as a means of bridging the theory–practice gap.

Educational facilitators are not the same as the former clinical teachers, who were based in the clinical setting but employed by the former schools of nursing. Educational facilitators, at least in local examples known to the author, tend to be employed by health-care trusts. Lecturer practitioners, in contrast, are invariably joint appointments, being employed jointly by universities and health-care trusts, spending an agreed quota of time in each setting. They have helped tremendously to give greater credence to the clinical element, along with the learning of practice in a higher education context. Providing the tensions inherent in being shared by two employers, albeit in partnership, can be resolved, this development should enhance the move to practice-based education. There remains a risk, nevertheless, that the lecturer practitioner may, at best, experience role conflict, and at worst, widen the theory–practice gap through a failure to reconcile what are still essentially different spheres. The lecturer practitioner's role should not be developed at the expense of underestimating the clinician's role in mentoring students.

It is notable that many studies of clinical supervision locate the nurse lecturer as the educator (Markham and Turner 1998, Severinsson 1998). In a similar vein Durgahee (1998), in his study of reflection on practice, cites the teacher in the classroom as the key agent, although reluctantly conceding: 'It is hoped that the findings could be used by teachers in a classroom setting and perhaps by clinicians in clinical practice while facilitating care'. Consultant nurses also represent a current feature of professionalization in mental health nursing, and through being closely linked to reflective practice, provide an illustration of the scope of the nurse as trainer in developing the facilitation of reflection on practice. It follows that emphasis in this examination should be with a view to evaluating Schon's (1983) concept in the professional development of practising nurses.

Mental health nurses, of all the health-care professions, have taken something of a lead in facilitating reflective practice. This sphere of training moves the trainee away from direct clinical practice and yet provides a very viable alternative to the dominant lecturing model that is encompassed in nursing's move into higher education, with the resultant overemphasis on theory. Reflection on practice, as derived from Schon's (1983) work, has in common with clinical supervision and preceptorship the role of mentor, named after the adviser to the young Telemachus in Homer's *Odyssey*. It is difficult to differentiate reflective practice from clinical supervision except that the latter is more formalized and indeed may be imposed upon clinicians by managerial directive. Reflective practice, in contrast, is more informal, perhaps in two specific ways: it is spontaneous, for example, it may provide the sequel to a critical incident in clinical practice. Moreover, it tends to emanate from the clinical level, by practitioners for practitioners, of their own volition. It tends not to be mandatory or part of a policy initiative. It is clearly distinct from didactic styles of teaching and learning. In effect, it involves the teacher, in Durgahee's (1998) words, 'moving from a sage on stage to a guide on the side'. Another interesting issue is whether reflection *on* practice (which for this purpose is synonymous with reflective practice) informs reflection *in* practice, i.e. the consciousness of doing something when one is actually doing it. Research is required so as to better understand these two distinct but related components of training. Perhaps through examining the importance of preceptorship, we can throw more light on this issue.

The advent of Project 2000 (UKCC 1986) brought with it the recognition that a bridge between the three-year course leading to the Diploma in Higher Education (Nursing) and the Registered Nurse role (RN) must be established. No longer could the former pattern of 'student one day and staff nurse the next' be allowed to persist. The attrition rate alone demanded that a more supportive environment had to be fostered for those making the transition. Thus preceptorship came to be a benchmark for advances in nurse education, largely due to the UKCC's guidelines that make preceptorship compulsory for the first four months of staff nurse experience (UKCC 1999, 2000). This optimum period is justified in that 45% of recent registrants felt confident after a period of between one and three months (UKCC 2000). In some cases this period has voluntarily been extended to six months and even one year. But what exactly is preceptorship?

The term 'precept' means a command or mandate; thus 'preceptor' indicates one who has authority over others, in a position of authority. By implication, therefore, the preceptor has control over the newly qualified Registered Nurse (Mental Health). This view is illuminated by the proposal to have three months supervised clinical practice at the end of the preregistration programme (UKCC 1999) to be continuous with the period of preceptorship. On the other hand, preceptorship is understood as student centred, whilst serving the newly qualified nurse as a precursor to PREP (Post Registration Education and Practice). It is somewhat ironic that by definition, clinical supervision, at least in the professional model from which it derives, suggests a more democratic dyad than does preceptorship, which by definition is conducted around a parental senior–subordinate relationship, in a practice context in which both participants have RN status in common. This suggestion of hierarchy is perhaps not the best platform for the promotion of lifelong learning, with its implications for partnership and sharing of skills, of which preceptorship is but the beginning.

The new developments in mental health nursing which emanate from pioneering work in other health-care professions could lead one to believe that there is now no place for the nurse as a role model. It would be erroneous to concentrate solely on such developments as clinical supervision, which essentially involves removal of the clinician from direct care, as a means of facilitating reflection. Role modelling, on the other hand, is an integral part of practice, such that those who practise together can learn together (ENB 2000). This is therefore an opportunity to examine the nurse as role model in the next section.

THE ROLE MODEL

The recent emphasis on the supervision model, a method that involves removal from direct client care, derives from a position that sees distance from practice, in temporal and spatial terms, as a prerequisite for reflection on that same practice. It is timely, therefore, to resurrect the notion that the nurse has much to contribute as an educator in terms of role modelling. This section therefore seeks to illuminate the great contribution that mental health nurses can make in demonstrating their skills to others. The argument for role modelling rests on the notion that mentorship incorporates much more than the emergent supervision model has tended to suggest. Student nurses have much to gain from direct observation of their mentor's expertise, as far as this is possible. Moreover, the role model's sphere of influence, or capacity to facilitate demonstration of skills, is too often overlooked and tends to be evident only when the nurse is drawn into 'critical incidents' (Flanagan 1954) or psychiatric emergencies, which may be, but are not necessarily, very public incidents.

Role modelling, in the context in which it is used here, is meant to indicate a planned activity rather than the spontaneous demonstration of skills evident in the kind of situations highlighted above. It is worth noting also that there is an inverse relationship between demonstration of skills and seniority in nursing. Evidence in relation to hospital-based care has consistently shown that the higher the grade of mental health nurse, the less contact they are likely to have with clients. There is reason to speculate that the same phenomenon occurs in the work of the community mental health nurse (CMHN), particularly in light of demands imposed by the Care Programme Approach, supervised registers (DoH 1994b) and the like. This attempt to look anew at the nurse's role as educator, and most particularly the nurse's discrete skills, act as a reminder that not only do mental health nurses lack the vocabulary to describe what they do, but additionally they fail to itemize particular skills that are largely unique and go some way towards constituting their distinctive clinician role. This is despite the fact that the interpersonal process model of mental health nursing (Peplau 1990) is eminently testable, according to Barker *et al.* (1997).

This section will try to redress this peculiar shortfall within the clinician's awareness of her own competencies, by dint of the comparatively recent development of reflective practice and the introduction of self-evaluation in practice assessment. Such an innovation goes some way towards providing a platform for future advances, by overcoming nurses' difficulties in conceptualizing their practice. Moreover, the generic tendency of mental health nurses will be examined in relation to linkage with other health and social care professionals. This is pertinent to the function of the nurse as a role model in that, in order to facilitate learning by demonstration of competencies, it is essential to understand what those competencies involve. Deciding at what level of learning these are situated is the most problematic of all the questions arising in this context. Insight into such competencies undoubtedly is a precursor to developing an identity and thus self-consciousness as a role model.

The mental health nurse is novel amongst the care professionals due to the greater exposure of the clinician to the client. In educational terms this can be exploited from within the care coordinator's role, so that a more effective use of resources is developed. Increasingly, this is a needs-led service, so if other disciplines can learn from the nurse, it is ultimately to the benefit of the client. The nurse as a CPA manager (NHSME 1996), for example, occupies a pivotal role in educating other carers. The nurse in stress management must be considered, as will the underlying practice paradigm which underpins the nurse as a model and thus an educator. Such an approach, it is hoped, will help shift attention from a current assessment-driven, supervision-led approach and give credence to a 'teaching by demonstration' approach once again.

Clinical practice has been shaped by a whole range of demands and conflicting loyalties. The latter is evidenced by *The Code of Professional Conduct* (UKCC 1992) which on the one hand underlines the primacy of the client as the nurse's major concern and fully endorses the possibility of the nurse serving as an advocate for the client, yet stresses that the nurse must cooperate with colleagues at all times, given the essence of nursing as teamwork. Whilst there is recognition that cooperation does not equate with collusion, it is also evident that advocacy and prioritization of the client's needs are not necessarily compatible with cooperation with colleagues.

The foregoing discussion points to the urgent need for a clear definition of mental health nursing which can somehow reconcile the inherent tensions within the role between the nurse as facilitator of human relatedness and the nurse as agent of social control. Barker and Jackson (1997) note the importance of what they call 'the new epidemics', namely depression, eating disorders and self-harm. They argue that no new services have been commissioned to address the needs of this diverse group of people which is expanding in proportion to the severely mentally ill, who, according to Barker and Jackson, are declining in numbers. Liaison with primary health care is seen as vital if the needs of this emergent group are to be addressed. Links with health visitors, district nurses and community workers will enable mental health nurses to be proactive. This is necessary if only because the problems faced by children at present, such as child sexual abuse, conduct disorders and general alienation, might well spearhead the development of personality disorders in those same individuals when they reach adulthood. Role blurring within a matrix of primary health care is presented as the necessary option, and has led to the emergence of the mental health worker (Sainsbury Centre for Mental Health 2000). If this means a more generic mental health nurse, then that is the way to go, argue Barker and Jackson (1997), if nurses are to lay claim to a needs-led service.

This is not to suggest that the nurse in mental health care has adopted a hybrid role in response to the prescription for multidisciplinary working (DoH 1996). Indeed, sound attempts are made to demonstrate the uniqueness of the mental health nurse's role and with it the resultant scope for modelling effective aspects of that uniqueness:

> ...being with and caring with people-in-care is the process which distinguishes nurses from all other health and social care disciplines, and needs to be recognized also as the process which underpins all psychiatric nursing. (Barker et al. 1997, pp. 660–667)

Nevertheless, it is reasonable to argue that the nurse as a role model in an educative role is stretched by an array of demands and, in effect, conflicting roles. By implication, such an experience of role conflict must come at a price:

> A feeling of being over-extended and exhausted does not necessarily imply that people are not coping with their work, but it is worrying, and people need to have adequate resources to do their jobs properly. (Open University 1997, p. 95)

It is in the role of care coordinator, rather than simply in the role of clinician, that nurses can demonstrate what they do best. Within the busy acute unit, for example, they have long had to interact with clients, relatives, doctors and other health-care professionals, sometimes all at once! It seems fair to suggest, therefore, that such a capacity for 'multitasking' is in itself a competency to be valued but one that has been grossly overlooked, being labelled by clinicians simply as 'administrative work'. Mental health nurses deserve credit for not only providing such a valuable resource but also demonstrating, by example, how to coordinate all the interested parties – and cope in the process! This again underlines the versatility of mental health nurses who have themselves so often dismissed such aptitudes as 'generic', particularly in relation to the current emphasis on specialist practice. This argument challenges attempts at overarching theory which seek to explain *the* reality of mental health nursing, rather than acknowledging *realities*. What is more, it shows nursing's adaptability; the nurse in mental health care can be interpreted as changing according to the client's requirements, rather than vice versa, as part of a move towards needs-led services. While it is difficult to say what mental health nursing is, we can say what it isn't: that is, it isn't a solitary activity. Effective professional care, even the most person-centred variety, involves two people, one of which is the nurse who, along with the client, is involved in a therapeutic relationship. Each needs the other, by definition, in a state of interdependency.

The concept of role model is derived from social skills training (Trower et al. 1978), in which demonstration by a confederate is intended to encourage the observer to benefit by what is called vicarious learning. This process involves the observer subsequently trying out the specific behaviour through role play in a psychologically safe training setting, before trying out the behaviour in the real setting. The problem with this paradigm in its application to nursing as a whole is that it is conscious; there is intention to demonstrate specific skills. Indeed, within the cognitive-behavioural approach, behaviours as well as cognitions are specified in order that everybody knows exactly what is going on.

The 'mainstream' of mental health nursing, on the other hand, is different in that much of the modelling effect happens spontaneously and is unplanned. The tradition of care coordination in the role of the mental health nurse is a key example. The nurse's collaboration with a range of other disciplines provides a platform for the demonstration of skills in working together within the clinical setting. Nurses can draw upon their role at the hub of health care to educate others. To practise active listening with the queries, anxieties and requests for information represents a central strand in the way forward towards greater openness and sharing of information and expertise. That nurses have coped with the often conflicting demands of quite diverse interest groups within the mental health-care setting is no little achievement. Through adopting the stance of being 'all things to all people' nurses have shown a marked aptitude for management of stress and as such present a highly credible example to other health-care professions, who tend to lack the experience of such a role and with it the expertise.

The liaison nurse presents an exemplary case as a role model to other disciplines in health and social care. It is an interesting development in mental health nursing and the liaison nurse as role model is positioned halfway between unplanned, spontaneous modelling and, at the other extreme, preplanned demonstration of how to conduct an assessment interview, for example. It is through links with the A&E department that, arguably, the liaison nurse has maximum impact.

People who harm themselves, particularly those who exhibit a regular pattern, have traditionally been given short shrift by some A&E staff, arising from their evaluation of worthiness in their patients. People who harm themselves are likely to be evaluated most negatively, as undeserving of care. The liaison nurse demonstrates competent communication skills and acts in a complementary way to the psychiatrist's role with people brought to the A&E department exhibiting self-harm. In so doing, the liaison nurse can actively challenge dangerous myths and misconceptions held around suicide, attempted suicide and self-harm, such as 'those who talk about it don't do it' which, as evidence consistently demonstrates, is a dangerous misconception (Fremouw *et al.* 1990).

It is important to note that the modelling effect, as a mechanism within social learning theory (Bandura 1977), is not contingent upon positive reinforcement. This means that a seasoned staff nurse does not have to gain any sense of reward when observing the liaison nurse adopting a non-judgemental approach, in order to move towards a more appropriate attitude as regards self-abusers, in line with that being demonstrated. This is not to suggest that clients who self-harm are easy to communicate with; on the contrary, they can be difficult people to help. It is thus not helpful to invest the liaison nurse with the role of expert. Rather, as evidence shows (Trower et al. 1978), the role model who copes, and is fallible, is likely to be most effective. The perfect model, if such a being exists, will teach by demonstration much less effectively, as observers are likely to perceive such a level of expertise as unachievable and thereby be deterred.

This is in contrast to the nurse as information giver. In this context the nurse as a trainer follows a more directive format, being seen as something of an expert. Yet it will become evident in the next section that such a distinction is not all that clear, owing to the fact that the role of the nurse as group facilitator lies at the intersection between education and therapy.

THE INFORMATION GIVER

Working in groups

In an educative role, the mental health nurse can be seen to operate in three specific groups: the anxiety management group, the problem-solving group and the social skills group. Anger management groups would slot into the same category, as would any self-help groups run on a practical basis. The distinction here is between 'talking' or support groups, on the one hand, and 'doing' or practice-based groups, on the other. It is the latter category of group work that will be emphasized in this section, related to the fact that education and therapy overlap so much, rendering attempts at classification very difficult. The perspective related to 'doing' groups will be examined in this section, along with the operational process which drives such groups. The expert/partner dichotomy must be examined in light of the image of information giving as 'like a lesson', thereby challenging the notion of the didactic teacher. Finally, the role of the nurse as information giver in the context of primary care will be highlighted as a marker of the future development of educational groups.

Groups which adopt a cognitive-behavioural approach focus on the 'here and now' in contrast to the psychodynamic approach which emphasizes early life experiences and how such experiences impact on adult life. The principle of anxiety management as an example of a 'doing' group often focuses on faulty learning in early development as an explanation of anxiety, but this emphasis is utilized as an opportunity to 'unlearn' problematic behaviour and adopt more adaptive responses. So, rather than fostering insight as a vehicle for change, information-giving groups seek to help participants execute change in themselves, through their own efforts, without recourse to much earlier traumas and repressed memories. Moreover, it should also be recognized that not all problems have a specific cause; phobic anxiety, for example, is not necessarily triggered by a noxious event but might have occurred spontaneously.

What of the nurse as a teacher in all this? A significant element of this approach, the educative function, is the didactic form in which the nurse as group leader gives practical advice, often to dispel any myths which the participants may hold. In terms of anxiety management, for example, there is a misconception that all anxiety is 'bad' or unproductive. However, it can be adaptive, even to the extent of preserving life, as the 'fight or flight' reaction (Cannon 1929) illustrates. Another common misconception held by clients is that nurses do not get anxious. Perpetuating such a myth has no therapeutic value, in that it is a misrepresentation of nurses as people and inveighs against the nurse being a coping model which, as mentioned earlier, has been found to be the most effective paradigm in helping others learn. This presents an opportunity to further explore the process evident in information-giving groups which extends beyond a mere information-giving strategy by the nurse, so as to enable the optimum degree of involvement of participants in their own group.

Much of what has been highlighted in this section would seem to point to the nurse as fulfilling the role of expert. This brings into focus the possibility of a tension involving two fundamental strands inherent in the current development of mental health nursing. On the one hand, the nurse as expert provides a springboard for professional advancement, particularly in terms of practice development (Allen 2000), with the nurse practitioner and consultant nurse at the hub of such advances. At the same time, nurses in general, and mental health nurses in particular, are active in fostering a partnership paradigm in the care setting. This trend is seen typically in the primary care sector, notably in the implementation of proposals that have centred primary care in the commissioning of services (DoH 1998a). Indeed, primary care groups (PCGs) have become prominent budget holders in the new developments and some have attained trust status (PHD 1998). The positioning of CMHNs in primary care places them at the interface with people reporting mild mental health problems, whose mental health needs can be met efficiently and expediently in the CMHN-led group such as that under discussion. By so doing, the nurse as educator is ideally positioned to inform people who, despite having no prior learning, wish to develop techniques in managing stress and anxiety.

Teaching people to calm themselves down serves as a reminder of (a) the importance of clients 'owning' their therapeutic group and its corollary, (b) the client as a partner in his care. The nurse should adopt a facilitative style. As

Carl Rogers (1983) proposes, people learn most effectively when they can choose what they learn. It is likely that clients will appreciate telling their own stories about their anxiety and such a strategy will enhance their feeling that it is a client-centred group, but only if it is positive and encourages change. 'Symptom swapping' as the sole feature of an anxiety management group is likely to jeopardize the integrity of the group, which suggests the facilitator will inevitably be in control of the session. If the nurse can offer her own reports this will position her as another human being rather than an omnipotent expert. Partnership in the role of educator requires that one is accessible and able to share some of the experiences of anxiety reported by clients. This is not to suggest, however, that the group become nurse centred. Rather, the successful educator will strike the right balance, enriching the group with her own self-disclosures of anxiety and yet at all times adopting an optimistic approach that rests on how she has coped with such feelings.

Nevertheless, the nurse as educator will require a knowledge base which can be brought into play when clarification is required, involving a more didactic approach. The nurse, for example, should guide group members towards a definition of the problem (or potential problem) of the individual concerned. By such means, the tendency towards abstraction, so evident in many psychothera-peutic support groups, is avoided. Challenging the many misconceptions about mental health provides another fundamental example of the need for infor-mation and can be explored at this point in the context of a problem-solving group.

Examples of misconceptions regarding mental health remain widespread and the nurse educator has a distinct role in challenging such beliefs. In so doing the nurse imparts important information to clients and the problem-solving group acts as a learning situation for all involved. 'You should pull yourself together!', 'It shows weakness to talk about your problems' and 'A real man doesn't cry!' are typical misconceptions that are perpetuated as cultural norms despite marked social change. The last example, for instance, flies in the face of reports of a greater willingness by men to talk about their feelings, although one study at least (Duncombe and Marsden 1993) finds no evidence of any such transfor-mation. What is apparent, nevertheless, is a greater readiness to seek counselling. Opposition to this trend, the 'we used to manage OK without counselling' school of thought, fails to consider the contemporary feminization of society in which masculinity of the 'tough it out' variety has lost much of its cultural capital.

The above illustration has relevance for the nurse's role as facilitator of infor-mation-giving groups in that all must be negotiated with clients in an ethos of equality. The nurse must not strive to always have the last word in a dominant style. Conversely, she should be able to cope without being too vulnerable, so as not to lose all credibility. There are risks involved, the most obvious being the self-disclosure involved in such groups in which the facilitator is expected to participate fully. It is recommended that the new inexperienced facilitator 'shadows' a more experienced facilitator, notably if she is undertaking preceptorship. Such measures concur with *The Code of Professional Conduct* (UKCC 1992) in which insufficient competency to undertake a specific intervention, due for example to lack of training, makes it the duty of the nurse concerned to report such a situation to her line manager.

Finally, it must be reiterated that the CMHN and community practice teacher are at the forefront of developments in primary care. The health centre setting, for example, will increasingly serve as a prime site for information giving. In such a way practitioners will have licence to inform the mentally healthy, those with mild mental health needs and possibly those people with severe mental health needs, although the latter group will be addressed more effectively in family settings, which will be covered in the next section. The waiting room, so long associated with tedium and with being an unproductive setting, can be transformed into a fertile site for running an ongoing 'defeating depression' ('beat the blues'?) or stress management group or perhaps an anger management group. A varied target group is on hand and such people could benefit from information giving 'going live' as a catalyst towards better mental health. Complementary to such groups or as an alternative, looped videos, as seen in so many museums and art galleries, could impart much information on mental health in the primary care setting and thereby could go some way to redress the imbalance in past policy developments such as *The Health of The Nation* (DoH 1994a) in which scant attention was paid to mental health (notwithstanding the targeting of mental health in *Our Healthier Nation* (DoH 1998a)). Mental health nurses should embrace the current trend towards public television viewing whilst in a pub or takeaway restaurant, using popular culture to project an accessible and acceptable message of mental health.

Family interventions

This educational context again involves working in groups; in this instance, however, a grouping that is found in all societies around the world: the family. Although a universal feature, the family, particularly in Western countries, has been held to be problematic and a key source of stress. Since Laing's pioneering work on the 'schizophrenogenic' family in the 1960s (Laing and Esterson 1964), the focus has moved away from pathologizing the family as a dysfunctional unit to the present, and far removed, position in which concern is centred on the rapid rise of suicide rates in certain social groups. This is largely a psychosocial focus, linked as it is to the notion of disengaged youth, and young males in particular. This picture of disadvantaged and disillusioned young men, alienated from both the family of origin and society as a whole, acts as a reminder that information giving within the family has much mileage in strategies aimed at preventing suicide, not least because of the anguished cry of bereaved parents: 'He didn't give any signs of being suicidal!'. It will be helpful, however, to acknowledge initially in this section the established role for family work in supporting clients with severe mental illness, revolving around the concept of high expressed emotion (Leff and Vaughn 1985). It is ironic, therefore, that the subsequent focus on young men in this section is associated primarily, according to commentators, with low expressed emotion in what is deemed to be, in a social context, a crisis of masculinity.

High expressed emotion is derived from the assumption that social environments, particularly intimate relationships and family contexts, are inherently stress inducing and, it is claimed, are associated in people living in such circumstances with a predisposition to schizophrenia. The capacity to cope with such stress is a measure of the individual's level of mental health. The tendency to actively retreat from overstimulation and become grossly withdrawn may be seen as indicative of severe mental health problems, namely the psychoses.

The concept of high expressed emotion is defined as involving critical comments, hostility and 'overinvolvement' (Rogers and Pilgrim 1996, p. 155). Dallos (1996) refers to 'psycho-education' being employed in such a setting. This approach aims to educate the family towards a more balanced level of emotional expression. They can be directly informed of the detrimental effects of an excessive degree of emotional expression, as demonstrated in research by Leff and Vaughn (1985), revealing that clients with schizophrenia are more likely to relapse if discharged to families with high expressed emotion. The nurse educator can contribute towards information giving by helping the family to examine the dynamics operating within their social unit. Moreover, information is given on the value of a problem-solving approach and the benefits of negotiation rather than confrontation, consensus rather than conflict, a reduction of an adverse family atmosphere and the benefits of boundary setting.

It will be apparent by now that information giving in such a setting is akin to family therapy; indeed, in both approaches the nurse is adopting an objective stance, observing family dynamics, viewing the family as a system, and at a suitable juncture can seek to feed back to the family what has been observed, whilst taking great care not to apportion blame in any way. The major difference is undoubtedly one of degree. Information giving will lean more towards directly educating family members of the actual and potential impact on the client if a high level of expressed emotion continues to persist. Another difficulty in definition concerns whether psychosocial family interventions are just that, interventions, or can best be regarded as education.

Notably, Droogan and Bannigan (1997) do not refer to education at all in their report of basing interventions in the families of people with schizophrenia. Citing a review on such interventions (Mulrow and Oxman 1997), they refer to the likelihood of success in reducing high expressed emotion. Moreover, the rate of relapse at 12, 18 and 24 months and additionally, admissions to hospital were reduced at both one year and over a period of 13–18 months. The overall picture becomes complicated by alternative evidence that low expressed emotion and understimulation can have just as damaging an effect (Brown and Wing 1962). It too can precipitate marked withdrawal and regression. This phenomenon represents the opposite pole from high expressed emotion and can now be placed in a contemporary context, in light of the grave concerns expressed in *Our Healthier Nation* (DoH 1998a) regarding suicide.

Rutter and Rutter (1992) argue that too much emphasis has been placed on the influence of the peer group in the socialization of adolescent males. They contend that the more concentrated environs of friendships are much more influential in the young man's development of gender identity and the problems around it. In contrast, conservative critics cite the highest ever rate of divorce and family breakdown and the steep rise in numbers of single mothers as the determinants of the crisis of masculinity currently being observed. Young men are identified at the centrepiece of such a trend and the steep increase in suicide rates of young men is seen as the primary indicator. In the past 20 years there has been a rise of 20–30% of men under 44 committing suicide, whereas in men over 44 a roughly equivalent drop over the same period has been observed (Office for National Statistics 1998).

Rather than contribute to this contentious debate, mental health nurses as educators would do well to concentrate on instituting information-giving strategies, if there is to be the remotest possibility of reducing the suicide rate of the overall population by 15%, as set in *Our Healthier Nation* (DoH 1998a). Given that another initiative, *The Independent Inquiry into Inequalities in Health* published later that same year (Stationery Office 1998), has made only broad recommendations with no specific interventions being proposed, this suggests this is an opportunity to redress the balance.

First of all, however, a note of caution is in order. It would be quite wrong to pathologize all adolescent experience as tantamount to mental health problems. As Benson and Cockerell (1997, p. 82) argue, it is essential that adolescent behaviour is seen within its sociocultural context so that unnecessary referral to mental health services is avoided and the most appropriate form of support is provided. The issue concerning adolescent suicide is convoluted further by the fact that a significant proportion of people committing suicide are not mentally ill. Notwithstanding such concerns, it might be useful to suggest information-giving strategies within the context of the family. This is not to position the nurse educator as a would-be health visitor but is an attempt to confront a tragic trend which sees youngsters, and males in particular, taking their own lives.

It is easy to fall into the trap of being prescriptive by advocating a singular style of parenting. As all modern parents well know, there is no fixed paradigm of parenting; rather, there is a plethora of strategies that can be brought into play if and when the need arises. There is much to support a youngster-centred approach to suicide prevention. Information to parents of adolescents should underline that speaking to them on their own terms is likely to be far more effective in encouraging young males to express their emotions. Their marked reluctance to do this is, of course, legendary and one can only speculate that continued gender-stereotypical behaviour in the form of 'laddishness' is a major explanation of the phenomenon. Education can serve as a major plank in suicide prevention. Nevertheless, such an approach might involve a radical change in the way communication, or the lack of it, is evident between parents and youngsters. The secret is for parents to be non-judgemental, just as it is in person-centred counselling (Rogers 1967). Such information giving thus has some evidence to support its application.

Moreover, it should never be assumed that everybody, including parents of the group under discussion, is aware of contemporary trends in suicide which might seem to mental health nurses to be common knowledge. Families may need to be told of the increase in young men's suicide, for example, in as clear and balanced a way as possible. In the face of such emotive concerns, it is unlikely that even the most rigid adherents of the 'toughen up' school will stick to their approach, particularly if their own son could be implicated. The presentation of such a sound rationale ensures that information giving is needs based, the youngster's need being to have hope for the future and a sense of self-worth. Mental health nurses, in their duty to care, owe our young people nothing less.

This is not to suggest that family interventions are the sole panacea for the nurse educator. Indeed, there is evidence that information giving is most effective with young people when it is delivered by people of their own age. This will become apparent in the secondary prevention section of the final part of this chapter, in which the nurse as educator in the realm of health promotion will be examined.

The health promoter

This point is an opportunity to outline the skills of the nurse as an educator in (a) prevention, particularly secondary and tertiary prevention, of mental illness (Caplan 1964) and (b) promotion of mental health, equated as it is with Caplan's primary level of prevention. The former requires competency in communicating with the individual, be it client or relative, and is akin to traditional mental health nursing, while the latter breaks from the orthodoxy, demanding public-speaking skills in which the nurse seeks out large audiences, given the practical difficulties of accessing non-clinical populations without imposing (unintended) negative labels and stigma upon them.

Caplan's model, serving as a milestone in relation to the nurse as an educator, will form the cornerstone of the remainder of this chapter. The three levels will dovetail with the sequential attention to the public as a whole, young men (Rogers and Pilgrim with Latham 1996) (in terms of promoting the expression of emotion), informal carers and finally the educator and service user groups, respectively, in a spirit of partnership rather than pedagogy.

PRIMARY PREVENTION

Prevention of mental illness

This requires an holistic approach, in which the nurse must take on board the social disadvantage shared by people with mental illness either, as is often common, in a premorbid state or, less commonly, social drift as experienced by middle-class people with long-standing mental health problems. By recognizing the social features germane to the prevention of mental illness, the nurse must observe for warning signs which can at least predispose to mental illness (Brown and Harris 1978). The nurse must equally be mindful of the expectation of an evidence-based approach. By so doing, she is able to draw from research findings in offering a rationale for primary prevention and the complexities therein. For example, Newton (1988) points to the complexity in detecting causative factors, asking: how do we know who is most at risk?

The answer is, of course, that we don't know at the present time, not least because of the absence of any single cause-and-effect relationship in the aetiology of the many mental health disorders that are, in themselves, extremely diverse. Instead, the best we can hope for is the detection of possible contributory factors, be these specific unplanned life events, lifespan transitions or social circumstances. This returns us to the need for a recognition of sociological factors. In appealing for a broader perspective, Rogers and Pilgrim (1996, p. 15) criticize Newton for following a medical model, in which she heads her chapters 'The prevention of depression' or 'The prevention of schizophrenia'. Their respondents, in contrast, repeatedly pointed to socioeconomic elements in terms of risk of mental illness, such as poverty, unemployment and poor housing (Rogers and Pilgrim 1996, p. 15). On the other hand, the need to prioritize resources, as highlighted by Newton, serves as a reminder of the impossibility of reaching everybody (when? who? where?), indeed all the disadvantaged, a large group as they are.

There is an argument for retreating to the level of the individual in preventing mental illness in the client himself, just as the medical model would have us do. Yet this social grouping, the socially disadvantaged, is noted for lacking an individual locus of control, with implications concerning their capacity for self-determination, so this is not such a simple issue. The best way through the impasse is to highlight what the nurse can do as an educator in both prevention and primarily through a health promotion initiative.

Promotion of mental health

Promotion of mental health can be traced back to the early 20th century, in the National Council for Mental Hygiene and the National Committee for Mental Hygiene, in the UK and USA respectively (Newton 1998, p. 11, Tudor 1996, p. 54). Such pioneering work has shaped the dual role of the present day mental health nurse in terms of prevention, akin to the medical model, as has the mental health movement which has largely opposed such a model.

The nurse as an educator should have some knowledge of models of health promotion, if only to better understand the complex dynamics likely to be involved in the process. For example, the health belief model (Redman 1993) is significant in that it warns against preaching a message that contravenes the cultural values of the group being targeted. An obvious example arises from the work of Rogers and Pilgrim with Latham (1996, p. 15) which found that a significant proportion of the population sought to resolve problems on their own and through their own efforts. This belief, underwritten by their valuing of self-help and independence, flies in the face of health professionals' tendency to celebrate counselling. In contrast, lay people can clearly be critical of such interventions brought in, for example, at times of great tragedy but sometimes contrary to the wishes of the relatives of victims of such tragedies.

Nevertheless, much has been achieved already by CMHNs, in particular, going into schools and disseminating more adaptive means of maintaining mental health. Guidance on anger management, stress management and communication skills, for example, helps equip youngsters to prepare for the world of work (and other aberrations of adult life!) whilst providing viable alternatives to smoking and substance misuse in general. It is the latter phenomenon that is causing the greatest concern and *Modernising Mental Health Services: safe, sound and supportive* (DoH 1998b), amongst other policy initiatives, documents the increasing link between substance misuse and mental illness. Providing resources are available and there is a will to enhance the nation's mental health, it is possible to envisage mental health promotion increasingly being conducted in the workplace and even in more unlikely settings: stress management for rail commuters is one example!

The nurse faces something of an ethical dilemma in seeking to walk a tightrope between people's rights to privacy and its association with self-help, on the one hand, and a duty of the nurse to enhance the well-being of the person with specific attention to mental health, on the other hand. Just as new policy proposals advocating assertive outreach to the severely mentally ill have implications for civil liberty, so too may mental health promotion developments impinge upon individuals' privacy, as evidenced by the findings of the above research study. Thus, it is *not* good to talk if it is manifestly against one's wishes. Having said that, it is time to dispel the Cinderella status of mental health care once and for all. For too long gross distortions, vast misunderstandings and unfounded mystique concerning mental health have been allowed to flourish unchecked. Providing the political will is there, the mental health nurse should act as a main player in fostering a more enlightened and informed attitude as befits this new millennium.

Comedy has often focused on mental health and mental illness as something of a 'soft target'. In 'Talent' (Newpalm Productions 1998), for example, a comedy written by Victoria Wood in the 1970s, the lead character refers to 'walking uphill in my flip-flops', claiming it is for the sake of her mental health! Journalists, on the other hand, often present much greater cause for concern. The so-called 'quality press' is no exception to such criticism. One article, for example, reports on a fan of the pop star Paul Young as '...writing from the asylum...' and asks 'Do you think she wrote it with one arm in and one arm out of the straitjacket, I ponder' (Lawrence 1998). The task of mental health promotion is daunting and will remain grossly underdeveloped (Rogers and Pilgrim 1996, p. 145) in the face of such damaging media reports.

The Mediawatch section of MIND is fighting something of a rearguard action in tackling such misrepresentations, not least, as Ramon (1998) argues, because other mental health pressure groups are responsible for some negative images in their campaign strategies. It is evident that widespread collaboration between interest groups is necessary if any effective campaign is to be implemented and the CMHN, in particular, is ideally suited to coordinate such community-based strategies. This is evident in secondary prevention as much as anywhere, as will now become apparent.

SECONDARY PREVENTION

Secondary prevention refers to the detection of early signs of mental illness (Caplan 1964). The nurse has considerable scope in educating key stakeholders on how to detect such signs. Noticing mild indications may be difficult for relatives as they may be too immersed in the emotional climate of the family to notice signs that can be transient and easily missed. One is thinking in particular of early clues to the onset of Alzheimer's disease, which may be little more than hints. Forgetfulness, for example, can be easily attributed to later life and is unlikely to cause any undue concern. A sudden change of personality, however, is unlikely to be overlooked by an informal carer, largely because such a sudden shift in behaviour can easily cause an emotional response in the 'significant other'.

In a family characterized by high expressed emotion, as has already been mentioned, it is difficult to envisage the fine discriminative skills required in detection, as the family is likely to be absorbed in their own adversarial and conflict-ridden atmosphere. In such instances, professionals are ideally placed for detection. Indeed, the trend currently is towards early intervention which, along with assertive outreach, is driven by *Modernising Mental Health Services: safe, sound and supportive* (DoH 1998b) and is geared towards accessing hard-to-reach clients.

The nurse educator has tremendous potential in secondary prevention, primarily through teaching relatives in general, and informal carers in particular, about the detection of likely signs that can act as an alarm bell, so that key agents of care can spring into action. One drawback is the likelihood of labelling and it would be unfortunate if informal carers adopted lay diagnostic procedure at the first sign of what is deemed to be a symptom. Clearly a previous history of a mental illness will inevitably act as a key determinant of detection, yet it is tempting to speculate that a greater emotional investment in *not* detecting early signs would be more probable. Further research is required urgently, as evidence about 'significant others' as detectors is not available, nor are there any apparent reports on outcomes from any such preventive strategies. Much of the shortfall derives from the low level of resources directed at preventive work by successive governments. To undertake secondary prevention is to enter uncharted waters.

On the other hand, earlier examples of recruiting relatives as co-workers are encouraging. As long ago as the 1970s, behaviour therapists were coopting relatives into the care process. The very same relatives had previously colluded with their spouses in the spouse's obsessive-compulsive behaviour and, most notably, agoraphobia. By educating relatives, they can be brought into a collaborative exercise in which all parties work together to enable the client to regain independence. This is only possible, of course, when there is complete support of the individual's recovery of coping levels and autonomy. Very rare but notable tragedies involving individuals manifesting 'the new epidemics' (Barker and Jackson 1997), yet hidden from the world, have pointed to a collusion in avoiding detection. According to Rogers and Pilgrim (1996) people much more readily access their GPs than go to a psychiatrist regarding mental health problems, attributable again to the fear of stigma, but it seems likely that CMHNs too are accessible, particularly if located in primary care. If so, the foundations are in place for nurses to train relatives to monitor closely the individual in question, be he a so-called 'revolving door' client or one with no previous access to mental health services.

This is not to suggest that 'significant others' are solely relatives. With the current concern around suicide in young men, it is incumbent upon the mental health nurse to recruit fellow youngsters into secondary prevention strategies, in schools, universities and workplaces. Adopting naturally occurring 'buddy systems' as ready-made support groups has a much sounder rationale than CMHNs struggling against the odds to gain rapport with young men in despair. As Rogers and Pilgrim with Latham (1996) argue, young people can communicate most effectively with young people, hence the need to coopt this group as co-counsellors in preventive initiatives.

As there is no automatic link between suicide and mental illness, this is an opportune point at which to examine the nurse educator's role in tertiary prevention, as it is at this level that the main thrust of prevention is focused upon people with more severe mental illness.

TERTIARY PREVENTION

Rogers and Pilgrim (1996, p. 154) define tertiary prevention as:

> ... *minimizing the impact of mental illnesses on patients' lives and preventing the 'relapse' of recurring disorders such as 'schizophrenia'... to identify, and if possible intervene in, the determinants of psychopathology, in order to minimize the probability of distress recurring.*

Put another way, the nurse can educate the client so that he can be helped to remain at his optimum level. As Rogers and Pilgrim (1996, p. 155) argue, there is little evidence that such approaches are adopted in contemporary psychiatric practice. On the other hand, current evidence suggests considerable advances in tertiary prevention aimed at people with long-term mental illness. Mental health nurses in general, and CMHNs in particular, are ideally positioned to take a leading role in such initiatives. By way of illustration, the potential for nurses to promote clients' own self-monitoring of symptoms should be considered.

It has long been customary to dismiss clients' own capabilities in tertiary prevention, yet recently Survivors Speak Out, a voluntary organization, has demonstrated that voice hearers can gain control over voices through their own efforts. Within the statutory services the emergence of cognitive-behavioural approaches for people with psychotic problems has demonstrated clearly that self-instruction techniques can be taught to clients. Equally, the self-monitoring incorporated into preventive strategies is a viable alternative to the omnipotent medical model. McDermott (1998) reports on a pilot scheme within Hounslow and Spelthorne Community and Mental Health NHS Trust in which clients carry a relapse record card along with a symptom thermometer, to be coordinated by CMHNs. The severity of illness of relevant clients is not clear but nevertheless this venture is emblematic of the challenges that lie ahead in the not-too-distant future.

It is in community mental health care that tertiary prevention comes to the fore. As mentioned in the reference to psychosocial family interventions, which are, by definition, synonymous with tertiary prevention, relapse rate is reduced, suggesting that early detection can have a marked effect on readmission rates. Furthermore, as Ness and Ryrie (1997) argue, statutory services cannot provide care for all referrals. This means that the CMHN is a key figure, in that she offers support to other care providers and, moreover, coordinates the many diverse agencies involved. This serves as a reminder that, as far as tertiary prevention is concerned, such collaboration can include clients and service user groups.

According to Butler and Rosenthal (1978), adults learn most effectively alongside other adults. Although such evidence is usually applied particularly to rehabilitation and resettlement in mental health care, it seems to be equally pertinent to tertiary prevention. In many respects the two terms are interchangeable. Tertiary prevention can be placed effectively in the sheltered workshop or the adult training centre, two settings that can make up a key feature of mental health care in the community, depending on the service provision, which ideally is determined by the needs of clients in the locality.

The nurse's role in this setting is threefold.

- The nurse tries to follow the principles of normalization, relating the work environment as closely to the community as a whole.
- Most importantly, however, the nurse can participate alongside the client. Mental health nurses have shifted from the role of 'doer' (Forster 1997), making the transition from 'doing for' to 'doing with' (Butler and Rosenthal 1978), the latter being the archetypal format for the nurse assisting clients with their resettlement into the community.
- Embedded in this role is tertiary prevention, in that the nurse is strategically located to prevent as far as possible further deterioration of the client and work routine has a vital part to lay in minimizing the impact of mental illness.

The nurse has a sound basis for building the relationship with the client: the nurse is partner to the client. Such a spirit of collaboration can form the bedrock for the CMHN in linking with service user groups.

The potential for service user groups to be involved in tertiary prevention has been demonstrated of late in The Netherlands. Client participation groups have developed within the last five years (de Wilde 1999) and education is included within their remit. The credibility of the clients is underpinned by their having had personal experience of mental illness. With training, clients can give advice, including at the tertiary level of prevention. Professionals can offer invaluable help, however, by bringing to the work a more systematic approach. Thus if separatist service user groups in the UK, such as Survivors Speak Out, are to work alongside mental health nurses, then they need to move away from their entirely collectivist activity, in which they have campaigned so effectively for reform, to more of a provider basis for the delivery of individualized care services. This would be similar to service provision already evident in the work of MIND. A reduction of the debilitating effects of mental illness has already been achieved by joint efforts. A prominent example is the training of ex-clients to become advocates for current clients. Successes such as these initiatives underscore the way forward as one of collaboration. With the slogan of 'let's work together', this positive pointer to the future provides an opportunity to summarize this chapter on the nurse as educator.

CONCLUSION

As the nurse education centre has shifted to the university, so too has training become education. This transition has seen a greater emphasis on academic study, such that nurse lecturers have surrendered their position in the practice setting. Yet this has been at a cost and demands something of a return to practice-based education. Practice is assessment-driven and will remain so and it is the nurse as a practice supervisor/mentor who is the trainer of student nurses. Yet the mental health nurse is not the passive recipient of delegated educational processes; amongst other achievements, nurses have led the emergence of reflective practice and, in particular, clinical supervision. Development of the nurse as educator in these areas, however, rests on the formalized support and guidance of lecturers, who are expected to be more active in practice placements in future.

Such is the emphasis on clinical supervision that the nurse has tended to lose sight of her many skills that can be directly observed. With the future of multi-disciplinary education looming, it seems a good time for nurses to highlight and demonstrate what they do, such skills often being unique. The difficulty for the mental health nurse has always been one of defining her role and this continues to jeopardize the nurse's impact as a role model. The act of information giving is, however, prominent in the role of the nurse as educator, demonstrating that clients can benefit as well as student nurses and fellow professionals. The nurse informs clients in both family and therapeutic group settings at a point where education and therapeutic interventions meet.

Health promotion is a neglected area in mental health care (Tudor 1996), and a range of policy developments have failed to commit the resources required to foster such developments. Much can be achieved by CMHNs going into schools and other such organizations to promote sound principles of mental health maintenance. Likewise, preventive measures can be directed at reducing mental illness, although there are marked difficulties in identifying vulnerable groups. Secondary prevention is similar to early interventions and prioritizes relapse recognition, strategies for which relatives can be recruited. A joint effort is essential in education, as the remit is so vast. At the tertiary level of prevention voluntary bodies and pressure groups can be drawn into a collaborative framework in order to redress the emphasis on reacting to tragedies in community mental health care, as highlighted in *Modernising Mental Health Services* (DoH 1998b). It must be emphasized that adopting strategies which are more preventive in their orientation requires a marked development in the role of nurse as educator.

REFERENCES

Allen, J. (2000) Stimulating evidence based nursing practice in the South London and Maudsley NHS Trust. *Netlink* 15: 8–9.

Bandura, A. (1977) *Social Learning Theory*. Prentice-Hall, Englewood Cliffs.

Barker, P. (1990) The conceptual basis of mental health nursing. *Nurse Education Today* 10: 339–348.

Barker, P. and Jackson, S. (1997) Mental health nursing: making it a primary concern. *Nursing Standard* 1(17): 39–41.

Barker, P., Reynolds, W. and Stevenson, C. (1997) The human science basis of psychiatric nursing: theory and practice. *Journal of Advanced Nursing* 25: 660–667.

Benner, P. (1984) *From Novice to Expert*. Addison Wesley, California.

Benson, A. and Cockerell, J. (1997) Sociocultural context of mental health nursing care. In: Thomas, B., Hardy, S. and Cutting, P. (Eds) *Stuart and Sundeen's Mental Health Nursing. Principles and Practice*. Mosby, London.

Brown, G. and Harris, T. (1978) *Social Origins of Depression: a study of psychiatric disorder in women*. Tavistock Publications, London.

Brown, G. and Wing, J.K. (1962) A comparative clinical and social survey of three mental hospitals. *Sociological Review Monograph* 5: 145–171.

Butler, R. and Rosenthal, E. (1978) *Behaviour and Rehabilitation*. J. Wright, London.

Cannon W. (1929) *Bodily Changes in Pain, Hunger, Fear and Rage*, 2nd end. Appleton, New York.

Caplan, G. (1964) *Principles of Preventive Psychiatry*. Basic Books, New York.

Dallos, R. (1996) Psychological approaches to mental health and distress. In: Hauer, T., Reynolds, J., Gomm, R. *et al.* (Eds) *Mental Health Matters*. Macmillan, Basingstoke.

de Wilde, G. (1999) *European perspectives of mental health and distress*. Seminar, Anglia Polytechnic University, Cambridge, 26 February.

Dexter, G. and Wash, M. (1995) *Psychiatric Nursing Skills. A patient-centred approach*. Chapman and Hall, London.

DoH (1994a) *The Health of the Nation*, 2nd edn. HMSO, London.

DoH (1994b) *Introduction of Supervision Registers for Mentally Ill People from 1st April 1994*. HSG(4)5. NHS Management Executive, London.

DoH (1996) *The National Health Service: a service with ambitions*. HMSO, London.

DoH (1998a) *Our Healthier Nation*. HMSO, London.

DoH (1998b) *Modernising Mental Health Services: safe, sound and supportive*. Department of Health, London.

DoH (1999a) *Making a Difference: strengthening the nursing, midwifery and health visiting contributions to health and health care*. Department of Health, London.

DoH (1999b) *The National Service Framework*. Department of Health, London.

DoH (2000) *The NHS Plan*. Department of Health, London.

Droogan, J. and Bannigan, K. (1997) A review of psychosocial family interventions for schizophrenia. *Nursing Times* 93(26): 46–47.

Duncombe, J.A. and Marsden, D. (1993) Love and intimacy: the gender division of emotion and emotion work. *Sociology* 27(2): 221–241.

Durgahee, T. (1998) Facilitating reflection: from sage on stage to a guide on the side. *Nurse Education Today* 18: 158–164.

ENB (2000) *Education in Focus: strengthening pre-registration nursing and midwifery education.* ENB, London.

Flanagan, J. (1954) The critical incident technique. *Psychological Bulletin* 51: 327–358.

Forster, S. (Ed.) (1997) *The A–Z of Community Mental Health Practice.* Stanley Thornes, Cheltenham.

Freidson, E. (1972) *The Profession of Medicine.* Dodd Mead, London.

Fremouw, W.J., Perczel, M. and Ellis, T.E. (1990) *Suicide Risk: assessment and response guidelines.* Pergamon Press, Oxford.

Haddock, J. (1997) Reflection in groups: contextual and theoretical considerations within nurse education and practice. *Nurse Education Today* 17: 381–385.

Knowles, M. (1990) *The Adult Learner: a neglected species,* 4th edn. Gulf, Houston.

Laing, R.D. and Esterson, A. (1964) *Sanity and Madness in the Family.* Penguin, Harmondsworth.

Lawrence, J. (1998) Farewell fame . . . but at least he's got one fan. *Independent* 13 March.

Leff, J. and Vaughn, C. (1985) *Expressed Emotion in Families: its significance for mental illness.* Guilford, New York.

Markham, V. and Turner, P. (1998) Implementing a system of structured clinical supervision with a group of Dip HE (Nursing) RMN students. *Nurse Education Today* 18: 32–35.

McDermott, G. (1998) Relapse: helping clients to recognise early signs. *Mental Health Nursing* 18(6): 22–23.

Milligan, F. (1998) Defining and assessing competence: the distraction of outcomes and the importance of educational process. *Nurse Education Today* 18: 273–280.

Mulrow, C.D. and Oxman, A.D. (1997) *Cochrane Collection Handbook.* Update Software, Oxford.

Ness, M. and Ryrie, I. (1997) A change for the better. *Nursing Times* 93(23): 36–39.

Newton, J. (1988) *Preventing Mental Illness.* Routledge and Kegan Paul, London.

NHSME (1996) *An Audit Pack for Monitoring the Care Programme Approach.* Department of Health, London.

Office for National Statistics (1998) *Mortality Statistics General Review of the Registrar General Deaths in England and Wales 1996.* HMSO, London.

Open University (1997) *Mental Health and Distress. Perspective and Practice.* OU Press, Milton Keynes.

Peplau, H. (1990) Interpersonal model: theoretical constructs, principles and general applications. In: Reynolds, W. and Cormack, D. (Eds) *Psychiatric Nursing: theory and practice.* Chapman and Hall, London.

PHD (1998) *Simple Guide to PCGs.* PHD, London.

Power, S. (1999) *Nursing Supervision: a guide for clinical practice.* Sage, London.

Ramon, S. (1998) *PhD research seminar.* Anglia Polytechnic University, Chelmsford, Essex, 17 September.

Redman, B. (1993) *The Process of Patient Education.* Mosby, St Louis.

Rogers, A. and Pilgrim, D. (1996) *Mental Health Policy in Britain. A critical introduction.* Macmillan, London.

Rogers, A. and Pilgrim, D. with Latham, M. (1996) *Understanding Mental Health.* HEA, London.

Rogers, C. (1967) *On Becoming a Person: a therapist's view of psychotherapy*, 2nd edn. Constable, London.

Rogers, C. (1983) *Freedom to learn for the 80's.* Macmillan, New York.

Rolfe, G. (1990) The role of clinical supervision in the education of student psychiatric nurses: a theoretical approach. *Nurse Education Today* 10: 193–197.

Rutter, M. and Rutter, M. (1992) *Developing Minds. Challenge and continuity across the lifespan.* Penguin, London.

Sainsbury Centre for Mental Health (1997) *Pulling Together.* Sainsbury Centre for Mental Health, London.

Sainsbury Centre for Mental Health (2000) *An Executive Briefing on the Implications of the NHS Plan for Mental Health Services.* Sainsbury Centre for Mental Health, London

Schon, D. (1983) *The Reflective Practitioner. How professionals think in action.* Harper Collins, London.

Severinsson, E. (1998) Bridging the gap between theory and practice: a supervision programme for nursing students. *Journal of Advanced Nursing* 27: 1269–1277.

Sharp, K. (1995) Sociology in nurse education: help or hindrance? *Nursing Times* 91(20); 34–37.

Stationery Office (1998) *Independent Inquiry into Inequalities in Health Report.* The Stationery Office, London.

Trower, P., Bryant, B. and Argyle, M. (1978) *Social Skills and Mental Health.* Methuen, London.

Tudor, K. (1996) *Mental Health Promotion.* Sage, London.

UKCC (1986) *Project 2000: a new preparation for practice.* UKCC, London.

UKCC (1992) *Code of Professional Conduct for the Nurse, Midwife and Health Visitor.* UKCC, London.

UKCC (1999) *Fitness for Practice.* UKCC, London.

UKCC (2000) *Standards for the Preparation of Teachers of Nursing, Midwifery and Health Visiting.* UKCC, London.

Wright, S., Elliott, M. and Scholefield, H. (1997) A networking approach to clinical supervision. *Nursing Standard* 11(18): 39–41.

4 THE NURSE AS THERAPIST AND COUNSELLOR

Doug MacInnes, Norman MacDonald and Matthew Morrissey

OBJECTIVES

After reading this chapter, you should be able to:

- understand the importance of the therapeutic relationship
- critically analyse your own skills in the formation and maintenance of the relationship
- demonstrate a knowledge of different therapeutic approaches and how they can be used with clients
- enhance your own practice under supervision
- define counselling as applied to mental health nursing
- show an increased awareness of the relevance of the use of counselling in mental health nursing
- demonstrate an understanding of counselling processes and principles
- demonstrate an understanding of counselling qualities and skills and their relevance in the work setting.

INTRODUCTION

Central to the work of nurses is what can be broadly described as therapeutic work. Such work initially needs an understanding of therapeutic relationships and an identification of ways to develop appropriate knowledge and skills as a practising therapist. This chapter will focus initially on the concept of the therapeutic relationship, since this is essential if further therapeutic, advanced work is to take place. Two approaches will then be discussed: the humanistic approach, which many nurses initially use, and then the cognitive-behavioural approach. We recognize that nurses will discover the way of therapeutic working which suits their personal style and this is to be encouraged as the nurse becomes more proficient. Throughout the chapter there will be clear references to practice so that the reader can link the theory to their own practice.

THERAPEUTIC RELATIONSHIPS

Therapeutic relationships skills are said to be essential to the practice of modern mental health nursing. However, there is still considerable debate as to how such skills are learned or developed. It is questioned whether we are born carers or whether we can learn skills such as how to build a therapeutic relationship.

Recently there has been evidence that the development of academic knowledge may take preference over the acquisition of basic communication skills essential for building therapeutic relationships. Research will be reviewed in order to establish whether the development of therapeutic relationships is based on science, art or magic.

Being with a person who truly and genuinely cares about you is a rare and priceless treasure. Perhaps the same could be said about therapeutic relationships in mental health care. Many nurses on acute psychiatric wards in the UK are under enormous stress to maintain standards of care. The reality, however, is that many have already lost this battle and many more will do so if provision for mental health services is not bolstered up in terms of investment in nursing care, given recent findings (Gulland 1998). Many people may lose sight of the fact that people with psychological problems need a range of support services including good nursing care and choice in regard to who cares for them.

A very fundamental aspect of care is building a therapeutic relationship. However, for a small minority of clients a therapeutic relationship is not always desirable or possible due to severe and recurrent criminal and frequently antisocial behaviour. There are real dangers for those who think that common sense or academic knowledge alone can prevent serious incidents. Nurses need significant experience and good therapeutic skills as a basis for learning effective interventions.

There needs to be trust, choice and reciprocity within any relationship for it to be called therapeutic. Being involved, sharing and listening can be rewarding for the nurse and client. However, there are signs that such basic aspects of developing therapeutic relationships may be left to junior or unqualified staff (Bradshaw 1998).

Of more concern is that nurses have to prioritize care such as various forms of observation to maintain the safety of clients. Such tasks create real pressures when qualified nurse numbers are low which often creates an environment of containment rather than being therapeutic. Some female clients have been assaulted while in mental health services, which can create further fears (MIND 1992). Nurses also have been assaulted in the course of their work (Ryan and Poster 1989) and yet continued to maintain a therapeutic relationship with the client who assaulted them.

Training for practice

Establishing a therapeutic relationship requires a certain level of trust and social skills which many people may find difficult, including student nurses. Users of mental health services require stable relationships with staff to have any hope of recovery. However, staffing levels are dangerously low in many acute services in London (Gulland 1998), apart from some specialist units. Mental health nursing students are often in clinical placements which are not ideal for them, other staff or clients.

One major concern is that a person with a mental health problem may get less therapeutic input in an acute service than if they were on a specialist forensic unit. The experiences of users of mental health services must underpin professional services and roles, where possible, in mental health (Heyman 1995). Yet we must also identify the safety and therapeutic needs of staff, particularly nurses. Building relationships is a skilled process which is fundamental to caring, mental health nursing and various forms of therapy.

Essential needs include accurate assessment and evaluation taking into account resistance to change at the level of the individual and the organization, and a clear relationship between theory and practice (Fielding and Llewelyn 1987). To enhance training effectiveness, recent studies indicate that clinical supervision can be therapeutic as feelings and concerns are ventilated as they relate to the educational process of learning within the nurse–client relationship.

What is a therapeutic relationship?

In mental health nursing a therapeutic relationship is defined as a relationship developed between two or more people essentially based on trust. In the practice of mental health nursing trust, caring and compassion have been rated highest in terms of qualities of the nurse–client relationship (Lowenberg 1994). The nurse–client relationship is the vehicle for the application of the nursing process and/or nursing models.

The goal of nursing care is to maximize the person's positive interactions with the environment, promote his level of wellness and enhance his degree of self-actualization. Through the establishment of a therapeutic nurse–client relationship and the use of the nursing process, the nurse strives to promote and maintain patient behaviour that contributes to integrating functioning. The basic building blocks are trust, warmth, genuineness and empathy which are referred to as *core skills* (Rogers 1961). A therapeutic relationship can provide emotional support, psychological comfort and learning (Davidson 1992, Smail 1978) and practical assistance. This is of course dependent on what nursing skills and resources are available. Such a relationship can have significant effects on helping the client and family to cope before, during and after a mental health problem.

What gives meaning to relationships is not always observable or measurable. The relationships with the therapist may be influenced by other past experiences or other relationships. Good relationships have been found to be integral to providing support for clients and carers, for example for individuals with manic depression (Hill *et al.* 1996, Morrissey 1998).

Not only do we need to develop a therapeutic relationship but we also need to be aware that there are different types. It has been suggested recently that there are essentially four types of nurse–client relationship:

- clinical relationship
- therapeutic relationship
- connected relationship
- overinvolved relationship

Although this is useful, there are other relationships that could be outlined including those which are abruptly terminated and being able to talk about impasses and failed therapies.

Being therapeutic

Some therapists see the relationship as the central factor in all of psychotherapy (Clarkson and Pokorny 1994). Kahn's teacher said, 'The relationship is the therapy' (Kahn 1991, p. 1).

Human relationships are important to some degree in all our lives. This has been well established for centuries and psychotherapy has no monopoly on that. Creating more harmonious relationships should be a central factor in developing our mental health services and society as a whole. Mental health nurses recognize that many clients have impoverished social networks and relationships (Blacker and Clare 1987). Being therapeutic is in part the creative use of self. Some would say it is a form of love – moderated love.

Kindness and compassion are essential. Other qualities are also important, like being friendly and having a sense of humour. Yet such qualities are not always present and may be seen as unnecessary extras by some professionals. Some would go as far as to say that therapy is bad for you (Masson 1988). While such debates are interesting, having a mental health problem requires skilled and often comforting assistance. For families and partners the emotional suffering is difficult to contain. Sadly, the condition known as schizophrenia can affect some individuals to such a degree that counselling and psychotherapy would neither be appropriate nor effective. The main reason is that schizophrenia is primarily neurochemical and no counselling or psychotherapy can reverse that fact.

It is also important to note that some clients would never be able to function in a psychotherapy setting but are still deserving of at least a therapeutic relationship. The therapeutic relationship is important in mental health nursing (Gournay 1995) and psychotherapy (Clarkson and Pokorny 1994).

Yet in practice, a day in an acute psychiatric ward illustrates many barriers to establishing either trust or engagement. These barriers include negative attitudes towards the mentally ill, staffing levels, the severity of psychological distress, changes in service provision, poor resources and lack of specialist services. There may also be an atmosphere of trying to maintain safety at the expense of personal freedom (Gulland 1998, MIND 1992).

Psychotherapy is available in psychiatric services but provision is often highly selective in terms of both clients and therapists. So on the one hand, the theory of psychotherapy suggests the importance of relationships but on the other, psychotherapy may only be available to a discrete selective sample who often have to pay for such relationships. Trying to establish such therapeutic relationships or alliances in practice poses serious dilemmas for mental health nurses given the current climate of psychiatric care (Gulland 1998).

More importantly, many nurses are aware of the need for developing good therapeutic relationships but may be restricted by the limitations of effective resources, leadership and effective nursing teams (Gulland 1998). Furthermore, measuring the therapeutic process continues to represent a challenge to many clinicians, including nurses, psychologists and psychotherapists. Therapeutic relationships are said to be a cornerstone of nursing and in particular mental health nursing. Clearly, for practising nurses, the basis and quality of such relationships varies significantly depending on the situation and the therapeutic style of the nurse or therapist.

Factors affecting the therapeutic relationship

Internal and external factors have a significant effect on the development of therapeutic skills and relationships. Some of the internal factors relate to the past experience and possibly fears of the student about engaging in group work, role play or other experiential work.

In some ways many students expect a checklist which they can use at once as part of the scientific model. Yet this is perhaps further affected by students themselves having difficulty with relationship skills outside the professional domain.

Trust is an essential aspect of any learning experience yet in reality students may feel threatened by classes which involve self-disclosure of any kind while ironically many clients are expected to confide in nurses their innermost feelings. Some organizational factors also may affect the building and maintenance of therapeutic relationships. Change is inevitable but it needs to be managed effectively. One of the damaging effects of the reorganization of services is that it breaks down teams, relationships and avenues of interpersonal support in the workplace. The stability of our emotional lives may be very much effected by such changes but stability is needed to work in mental health services with people who have emotional and psychological problems.

Learning how to develop therapeutic relationships continues to remain a contentious issue in the education and practice of not just mental health nurses but also doctors, clinical psychologists and other health professionals. At a macro level there is still a very broad debate on what a therapeutic relationship is and how it is constructed. A more important question is whether such skills are innate or learned.

In science there is a focus on gathering data, measuring, generating hypotheses and developing new theories. Although very seductive, the issue of measurement may be severely flawed in the main due to the complex nature of our social relationships. However, there has been intense interest in this topic in nursing (Peplau 1952) and psychology (Katayama 1997, Morse et al. 1997). Much of the research has focused on the dynamics (Forchuk 1994) and models (Morse et al. 1997) in relation to nurse education (Katayama 1997) and challenges to recent assertions regarding the purpose of nurse–patient relationships (Chinn 1997).

Although there are many studies on therapeutic relationships, many echo the basic building blocks of developing a therapeutic relationship, establishing a trusting relationship and core skills in regard to empathy and client-centred approaches. Recently it has been suggested that comfort is the basis of therapeutic relationships (Morse et al. 1997) based on ideas originally put forward by

Smail (1978). This model has not gone uncriticized (Chinn 1997). The main challenge was on the definition of comfort yet in reality discomfort can also bring about change and not necessarily break the therapeutic relationship. However, for this to happen the client must have a good knowledge of and trust in the nurse.

Students and clients may feel far from comfortable with interactions and power is an important issue for all which may not be addressed by clinicians or educationalists. More importantly, students may have very limited exposure to either role play or direct clinical experience and supervision (Pieranunzi 197). It is clear that those involved in training mental health nurses must be sensitive to the learning needs of students.

Learning to build a therapeutic relationship

Learning how to build therapeutic relationships is viewed as basic to all forms of nursing (Peplau 1952). However, this ingredient of care, which is often developed while attending to basic nursing needs, is often delegated to nursing assistants (Bradshaw 1998). Yet in reality such skills are the hallmark of all nurses, particularly mental health nurses. To date there is little research evidence to show whether therapeutic skills can be easily learned in the classroom (Katayama 1997), are effectively assessed or measured, are effectively supervised in practice or are truly valued. It would be difficult to show how a person develops therapeutic relationships but we do know that practice and feedback are important.

After qualifying, many nurses end up compromising their values in order to get on with colleagues. However, it is important that a student can become proficient and understand the importance and nature of therapeutic relationships. One way to help the student learn is to use a simulator which is made up of video clips. For example, a student can watch a video clip of a distressed client and listen to different responses from her nurse. The user can select the response that seems right, listen to an experts opinion of the selection and then list to the patient's reaction to the selection. Many conversations between client and nurse are possible. There is also a quiz using this programme. Case studies and feedback and assessment with a clinical supervisor are other methods available to enhance understanding and learning around being therapeutic.

The experience of some student nurses illustrate the difficulties in coming to terms with developing a therapeutic relationship, as part of the nurse–patient interaction, as can be seen in the following statements.

How do I know what to say and what not to say? (Student)

It's hard to say when a therapeutic relationship develops and I'm not really sure anyone ever tells you that you have done it right, it's really got to do with gaining experience, recognizing that people are not like what is described in textbooks. (Student)

As a student on placement you often struggle with your own confidence so I think it's hard to be relaxed, not to mention being therapeutic. (Student)

Some students say they are really scared of upsetting patients but I think what's the point in that as most patients can sense things like that. I don't think you can teach someone how to be genuine, you either are or you're not. (Student)

Looking back I suppose I had great expectations. As a qualified nurse I would say the most therapeutic thing I do is to chat and watch television with the residents. Giving a compliment can be a big thing for one of the residents only if they value you and your opinion. Yes, liking each other is part of what makes a therapeutic relationship but respect is much more important. (Staff nurse)

The above experiences are part of an ongoing research project which demonstrates some of the issues surrounding difficulties students may experience in learning about therapeutic relationships. For many students a positive relationship with a college tutor can be the first significant experience of respect, genuineness and trust for the student.

However, therapeutic skills are not simply developed overnight. We are continuously learning about our relationships. Teaching surrounding this topic needs to appreciate the process and the skills involved in developing and maintaining therapeutic relationships. Clearly any theoretical model must be related to practice with examples. Individual components of knowledge and skills must be broken down and include practical and clear feedback to the student. The simple practice model shown in Figure 4.1 is based on the idea that the student learns best from coaching and clear feedback. The stages of skill acquisition can be used to guide the student, with supervision and tutorials as forms of support.

In order to learn therapeutic skills in practice, student nurses need to have an identified clinical supervisor. The link tutor can also arrange meetings to ensure that learning experiences are available and that clinical supervision takes place and is monitored. The learning loop identifies a starting point for each student. Although the student may have covered the theory in the classroom such knowledge may need to be reactivated in practice. Coaching skills are needed by the supervisor and the link tutor, which should not be presumed because of formal qualifications. Then follows rehearsal where the student is sometimes reassured by the supervisor and in some cases by the link tutor. However, feedback is the most essential element of this process and perhaps often overlooked. The acquisition of the skill is the next stage but is reinforced by preparation, delivery and peer evaluation.

It is debatable whether the therapeutic relationship can be broken down into a science or an art. However, when an experienced mental health nurse establishes a therapeutic relationship which is based on trust, warmth and genuineness, the results, though sometimes not apparent, are nevertheless magical and comforting.

In the next section various therapeutic approaches will be explored using case studies to demonstrate different ways of working with clients.

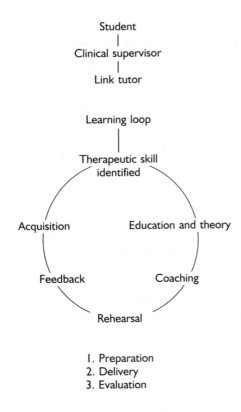

Student
|
Clinical supervisor
|
Link tutor

Learning loop
|
Therapeutic skill
identified

Acquisition

Education and theory

Feedback

Coaching

Rehearsal

1. Preparation
2. Delivery
3. Evaluation

Figure 4.1   Therapeutic Skills Practice Model (Morrissey, in press)

HUMANISTIC COUNSELLING

Introduction

Counselling is not one approach or therapy and can mean many things. Like the term 'therapy' itself, counselling is a notion that is inescapable in the world of nursing, particularly mental health nursing. It appears in specific contexts, for example bereavement counselling or AIDS counselling, but also in less well-defined areas, for example supportive counselling, and it even has unfortunate associations with disciplinary processes, for example in terms of counselling someone about their lateness. Counselling can be undertaken with individuals, couples, families and groups. The counsellor might be someone who professionally does nothing else or it might be seen as one part of a job of work, as it is most often in the field of mental health nursing. The theoretical underpinning might be analytical, cognitive or humanistic and within each of those there is a range of models and associated processes, principles, qualities and skills.

It is important therefore to establish a working definition of perhaps the most helpful counselling approach in mental health nursing, while acknowledging that this is but one of many and cannot be universally applied. In counselling literature, a wide range of terms is used; for example, 'therapist', 'counsellor', 'helper', 'facilitator', 'patient' and 'helpee'. For the sake of convenience, the terms 'nurse' or 'she' and 'client' or 'he' will be used here.

In the context of mental health nursing, humanistic or client-centred counselling is essentially a process in which the nurse offers the client time, space and skills to help him see the nature of his difficulties more clearly and decide on the direction in which he should go. The approach is based on the work of Carl Rogers (1961) and more recently Gerald Egan (1994), although many others have described models consistent with theirs, albeit with some variations. While some specialist nurses are able to apply the work of these writers to the letter, most nurses are rarely counsellors in the sense that they have had specialized counselling training and devote their entire professional time to counselling. Such professional counsellors will work largely on an appointment system, with the client requesting help for a specific difficulty or being referred by another professional agency for a specific purpose. However, mental health nurses in any setting are in a position to use counselling skills and principles in their work with patients and their relatives, colleagues and junior staff.

In mental health nursing, the client might be a patient on a ward who needs to talk about his redundancy, which appears to be an important factor in his depression. The client might be a junior member of staff, who asks if he can 'have a word in private' about something that is bothering him. The client might be a patient's relative who is in some distress about how they are going to cope when the patient is discharged. The client might be a person referred to a community psychiatric nurse (CPN) because he has problems controlling his temper. In all these cases, the nurse is in a position to use counselling skills, such as active listening, rapport building and problem solving and to demonstrate the qualities associated with counselling, such as empathy, non-judgemental acceptance and unconditional positive regard.

The nurse should have a framework to base her work on, to avoid losing all sense of direction (Barker 1989, Burnard 1994, Egan 1994, Ivey 1988). It is important to remember, however, that client-centred counselling is only one approach to working with people in a therapeutic or helpful manner. It is not a cure for all ills and indeed is not always appropriate. For example, the client might be unable to make reasoned informed decisions, perhaps because of an acutely confused state, or there may be a need for some form of physical intervention, perhaps to relieve acute distress or for safety reasons. Nevertheless, the principles, skills, qualities and frameworks of counselling are central to mental health nursing and may be used with the majority of clients. These issues and their implications will be explored below.

Counselling principles

The central principle of humanistic counselling is that the person who knows best is the client. The client after all is the only one who knows about his own personal world, values and attitudes. He alone has intimate knowledge of the people important to him and of the events that may have contributed to his problems. He alone knows which potential solutions to his problems are realistic and acceptable. The nurse does not live in the client's world and can only work with, rather than work on, the client. The client has both the right and the responsibility to make his own decisions and the role of the nurse is to help him to look at his own position and make decisions about what he wants to do, whether that be to accept the position or to change the position in some way. For example, in a bereavement problem, it might be more appropriate to move towards accepting the situation, whereas if the problem is related to a current relationship it may be best to look at ways of changing behaviour, perhaps in the way in which feelings are shown. At times the focus should be on adjusting the emotional response and at others on adjusting the situation itself but the things to be explored and the decisions on how to address the situation must be controlled by the client.

One of the classic assumptions about counselling is that it involves giving advice to the client. The very word 'counsel' used to mean 'advice' and is still used that way in the context of working with lawyers. However, giving advice in mental health nursing is fraught with difficulties, if not danger. Indeed, Morrison and Burnard (1991) suggest that the client-centred approach is the very opposite of advice giving. Advice is recognizable by words like 'If I were you . . .' or 'What you ought to do is –'. Such advice may be judged to be appropriate or inappropriate, and the client may choose to take it or leave it but none of these combinations is ideal. If the advice is appropriate and the client takes it, then there is a positive outcome, except for the fact that the client has learned to be dependent on the nurse for making decisions, moving towards the idea of 'learned helplessness' (Seligman 1973), which in the long term is very far from being in the best interest of the client. He has learned that the way to solve problems is to ask the nurse. If the advice is appropriate and the client chooses not to take it, then the therapeutic relationship is adversely affected. If the advice is inappropriate and the client takes it, then there is clearly a poor outcome. Finally, if the advice is inappropriate and the client chooses not to take it, then it would seem that the client would have been better off without the nurse's advice in the first place. In any case, what might be appropriate for one client or what might have been helpful personally for the nurse in a similar situation might not be the best for the client at the time. Giving advice in the context of mental health nursing is clearly far from the ideal approach.

There is, however, a nice but important distinction between giving advice and giving information. Solving a problem for a client is very different from helping them to solve it. Part of helping him in that process might be teaching or working with him using a specific problem-solving strategy. Giving information is part of empowering the client, where making decisions for them is quite the opposite. An example of giving information might be telling the client that, following the loss of a close relative, it is quite common for the bereaved to feel as though the deceased were in the room with them. Such information might reassure the client that he is not going mad, whether or not he acknowledges to the nurse that he has had that experience. Another example is that issues of what is and what is not 'safe sex' should be more in the vein of information giving rather than making moral demands on the client. Telling him facts is very different from telling him what he should or should not do. The client should remain in charge and responsible for his decisions and actions.

Counselling qualities

The qualities of the mental health nurse in the context of counselling are in a way a bridge between the principles of counselling and the specific skills used by the nurse. The principles are related to the context and aims of the work undertaken and the skills are of course the techniques used to achieve the aims. The qualities are related to the attitudes or attributes of the nurse but to be effective these must be demonstrated by the nurse, which requires communication skills. Principles, skills and qualities are quite different but inextricably linked.

Different theorists have described different qualities essential to counselling but the issues which recur regularly are empathy, positive regard, respect, concreteness, immediacy and non-judgemental acceptance (Ivey 1988). Each of these qualities can be viewed as private or public and both aspects must be considered.

Empathy

There are many definitions of empathy (Alligood 1992, Baillie 1996, Gould 1990) but it is generally accepted to be the nurse understanding the world from the client's point of view: being on the same wavelength but remaining objective rather than getting overinvolved or appreciating the client's distress without herself becoming distressed by identifying with that distress. This should be distinguished from the other '-pathies', namely sympathy, apathy, antipathy and compathy.

- *Sympathy* is identifying with the client's distress and being as emotional about the situation as he is.
- *Apathy* is being indifferent to the client.
- *Antipathy* is being pleased that the client is in distress.
- *Compathy* is developing similar physical symptoms to the client (Morse and Mitcham 1997).

These might be internal experiences, in that they are what the nurse feels and not necessarily what the nurse shows, but the associated behaviours are important to acknowledge. These behaviours might be illustrated by the metaphor of the nurse being in a rowing boat, seeing someone in the water, waving their arms in distress.

- the *sympathetic* nurse would panic and possibly throw herself into the water.
- the *apathetic* nurse would just row past.

- the *antipathetic* nurse would laugh and row away.
- the *compathic* nurse would shiver and gasp for air.
- the *empathic* nurse would row over to the person and help him into the boat.

There is no doubt which is most helpful.

Empathy has been described as being with the other person but knowing that you are not them (Zderad 1969) and the ability to understand another's world accurately and to respond so that they feel understood (Nelson-Jones 1986). While empathy therefore implies a degree of compassion and sensitivity, empathic listening requires two types of communication skill:

- the ability to listen and observe with care and accuracy
- the ability to convey understanding to the other person.

Listening and observing with care and accuracy, focusing attention fully on another person, involves a conscious decision. Given pressure of work and the distractions that occur, both internal and external, it is not always easy to 'clear a space' for the other person (Gendlin 1981). A decision must be made to give time totally and exclusively for a while – the conscious use of self (Heron 1977). Empathy is impossible without full concentration on the client. Egan specifically suggested five non-verbal strategies that would help the client feel that full attention was being paid to him, with the acronym SOLER.

- sit Squarely to the client
- maintain an Open posture
- Lean slightly forward
- use appropriate Eye contact
- stay Relaxed (Egan 1994)

This implies that the nurse always has control over the environment where the session takes place, which is not always the case when visiting someone's home. Cultural differences must also be taken into account; for example, in some cultures looking directly into someone's eyes is considered to be disrespectful. Nevertheless, Egan acknowledges the importance of the non-verbal aspects of behaviour, particularly when establishing rapport or attempting to show that the nurse is focusing completely on the client. This has been described as 'total listening' by McKay (1983) who, in addition to non-verbal behaviour, suggests that the nurse might reinforce the client by nodding or paraphrasing, seeking clarification, asking questions, actively moving away from distractions and being committed, even if angry or upset, to understanding what was said.

Demonstration of understanding requires focusing on the 'feeling content' as much, if not more, than the 'fact content' of the client's verbal and non-verbal behaviour. By reflecting feeling, the nurse shows that she is trying to understand the way the client sees things, as well as checking the accuracy of her perception. For example, even though the client might not have talked specifically about his feelings about a subject, the nurse may have been sensitive to the emotional content and might say 'So your boss's attitude makes you feel frustrated'. This can also help the client to focus on his feelings, enabling him to deal more effectively with them (Authier 1986). It may be appropriate to combine reflecting feeling with paraphrasing the factual content of what the client has said, for example 'So your partner told you to get out, and you seem quite confused about what to do now'. Making statements rather than asking questions also gives the client the choice of whether or not to say anything further.

Specific techniques for developing rapport and showing empathy might therefore include the following.

- *Showing that you are listening*: give non-verbal signals by alert posture, appropriate gaze, nodding, smiling or minimal encouragers such as 'mm', 'I see', 'Yes'.
- *Being aware of the total content of the message*: listen to what is being said, but also pay attention to the way in which it is being said, which gives clues to the client's emotional state.
- *Listening for cues*: be aware of key words or themes that may be repeated by the client, particularly those suggesting hopelessness or no view of the future, which might indicate suicide risk.
- *Looking out for incongruence*: the words might convey a different meaning from the way in which they are spoken. For example, someone might say 'I'm fine' when all the non-verbal behaviour and the tone of voice suggest otherwise.
- *Using silences effectively*: allow the client time to reflect on what has been said or what he is going to say next. Although it is certainly not the case that the longer the silence, the more therapeutic it is, you should avoid the temptation to fill silences to relieve your own anxiety or move on too quickly.
- *Using appropriate language*: avoid jargon or being condescending. The client's social, cultural and educational background should be considered.
- *Reflecting level as well as type of feeling*: there is an important difference between being 'furious' and being 'irritated', for example.
- *Reflecting appropriately*: sometimes feelings can be effectively acknowledged by silence and nodding rather than by trying to put feelings into words.
- *Paraphrasing appropriately*: putting the client's material into your words can help clarify issues, as well as showing that you understand.
- *Summarizing appropriately*: going over what has been said or discussed can help the client see things from a different perspective, as well as lead on to a plan for further discussion or action. It is also a good technique if you are yourself uncertain which avenue to explore next.
- *Saying as little as possible*: it is important to remember that the client is the most important contributor in the session.

Positive regard
Positive regard involves focusing on the positive attributes or behaviour of the client, although he himself might be viewing things in a negative light. It requires

the ability to notice, attend to and value attributes that the client himself might find difficult to acknowledge. A typical example might be the depressed person who feels he is unable to do anything and the nurse could observe that, given the tremendous effort involved, his attempt at describing the problem represents a great achievement for him. Someone who abuses alcohol at times might feel guilty or full of remorse, and, while accepting that those feelings are real and distressing, the nurse could acknowledge his ability to resist alcohol at times or give positive feedback on his efforts to find other coping strategies.

Respect

Closely associated with positive regard is the notion of respect and warmth. Harre (in Egan 1990, p. 65) argues that the deepest human need is the need for respect – being valued as a human being. For the nurse to demonstrate respect, she should encourage the client to find his own way through his difficulties, searching for a solution that suits him, which may not necessarily be a solution that the nurse would have chosen in a similar situation. The nurse should treat the client as a unique individual and not impose her own values or standard solutions.

This is closely related to the idea of non-judgemental acceptance, described below, but can also be shown in very unsophisticated ways, such as being available for the client rather than avoiding him and being reliable in terms of keeping to arrangements for working with the client, even in such basic things as turning up on time.

Non-judgemental acceptance

One of the essential features of the client-centred approach is that the client needs to know that, whatever the nurse's feelings about who or what he is or what he has or has not done, he is accepted for what he is (Murgatroyd 1986). Non-judgemental acceptance is the nurse's ability to suspend her own opinions and attitudes and take on a 'value neutrality' towards the client (Ivey 1988, p. 131). The idea is closely related to the qualities of positive regard and respect and can be shown by tone of voice and body language, as well as by statements that indicate neither approval nor disapproval of the client's position, beliefs or actions.

While this is undoubtedly desirable, it may prove more difficult to achieve or demonstrate than some of the other qualities, since it often happens that someone working through difficulties believes something quite different from the nurse's own beliefs or has done something of which the nurse disapproves. For example, a client might be concerned about being pregnant and the nurse might have different beliefs about termination; a client might admit to having been violent towards his children in the past, which the nurse might find outrageous; or he might have doubts about a forthcoming arranged marriage, a concept quite alien to the nurse. In such cases the nurse's own beliefs or experience could quite naturally influence her response to the client.

Non-judgemental acceptance does not require the nurse to be indifferent towards important issues but rather to listen to the client carefully to try to understand his point of view or actions. The focus should be trying to understand the client, not making judgements on his beliefs or morality. Rogers (1967, p. 102) describes 'unconditional positive regard' as communicating to the client a genuine caring, not affected by subjective evaluations of his thoughts, feelings or behaviour. For example, a former drug dealer concerned about his ability to maintain relationships should be viewed as a person with interpersonal problems, not as someone evil who deserves to be alone because of past actions.

It is, however, idealistic to think that the nurse will always be able to set personal feelings, attitudes or beliefs aside. She may feel so strongly about something (for example, that someone with a history of sexually abusing children should be punished rather than treated) that she is not able to work effectively or positively with such a client. In such circumstances it would be appropriate to acknowledge this and possibly for someone less affected by the client's history to work with him. The fact that the nurse feels strongly is not wrong or professionally imperfect but it is important for both the nurse and the client that the feelings are acknowledged rather than denied. Clinical supervision is one way in which the nurse may be helped to identify and explore such issues.

Concreteness
Concreteness refers to both a quality or set of attitudes and certain helping behaviours. It is concerned with being specific rather than vague or general and as well as helping the client to clarify his own thinking, it shows that the nurse is interested in finding out more about what is going on in the unique world of the client. For example, if a client says that he 'can't cope with pressures', the nurse might ask for examples of relevant situations and for some detail of what exactly happened in terms of the client's thoughts, feelings or behaviour. If another says that he is 'depressed', then the nurse might ask how that depression affects him, perhaps in his view of the future, patterns of eating and sleeping or whatever. Clearly the client should not be bombarded with questions as though being interrogated but it is important that the nurse avoids jumping to conclusions and asking for detail or clarification can also show interest in working with him as an individual.

Immediacy
The notion of immediacy is related to the idea that it is often appropriate to focus on the present rather than dwell on the past and particularly on the actual relationship between the client and the nurse and how that might reflect other relationship issues for the client. For example, the nurse might say that she notices that the client seems to find it difficult to trust her and ask whether this is something to do with her or if this is generally the case for the client. She might notice that the discussion is not going anywhere and suggest that they stop for a moment and look at why things are not progressing. She might point out that the client looks particularly agitated or angry.

Immediacy requires the nurse to be aware of emotional and relationship issues in the discussion as well as giving attention to the factual content. Egan (1990, p. 229) suggests that immediacy can help the nurse and client work together more effectively and that what clients learn about themselves in their work with the nurse can provide new perspectives on how they related to people in their everyday lives.

The counselling process

Counselling as a process involves certain stages, from the first meeting between the client and nurse through various activities to the final meeting. It is certainly important to have a model or framework within which to operate; Barker (1989) uses the analogy of the importance of having a raft, in order to avoid drowning in a 'sea of possibilities'. Different writers divide the process into different numbers of stages or steps; for example, Stewart (1983) has nine, Egan (1990) three, Ivey (1988) five and so on. Culley (1992) simply labels her three stages the beginning, middle and end. Irrespective of the numbering or labelling, the writers tend to agree on the general sequence the work should follow.

First, it is essential to establish a working relationship with the client. This involves developing rapport and agreeing the nature of the work in terms of boundaries, confidentiality and so on. It is obviously important to start on the same wavelength as far as possible. The client is then helped to define and explore the problems or difficulties – to tell as much about his situation as is necessary. Once the problems have been defined, the client is helped to look for and at alternative ways of dealing with them, typically either by changing the situation or by changing the way he looks at it. The nurse then helps the client to commit himself to ways of achieving his goals and to put the plan into action.

The key word throughout the process is 'help'. The nurse works with the client on solving the problems, rather than solving his problems for him. In order to achieve this effectively, she needs different skills at different stages of the process. Initially, during the rapport building, she will find listening and probing skills particularly helpful. Saying as little as possible, using active listening techniques and minimal questioning will enable the client to tell his story in his own way – reflecting feelings and paraphrasing will show that the nurse is interested and paying attention. There must be some flexibility about the topics covered and the order of covering them; rather than using a preset order of prepared questions, a more natural conversational style will help put the client at ease (Brown 1995), as well as allowing him to stay in charge of the agenda.

COGNITIVE-BEHAVIOURAL THERAPY

Cognitive behavioural therapy (CBT) is a generic term referring to therapies that incorporate *behavioural* interventions, which are direct interventions to reduce dysfunctional emotions and behaviour through altering behaviour, and *cognitive* interventions, which attempt to reduce dysfunctional emotions and behaviour by altering individual appraisals and thinking patterns. Although these treatments are derived from the theoretical concepts that underpin behaviour therapy, Brewin (1996) noted the differences between the two treatment models. Behaviour therapy is based on the assumption that actions and emotions are under the control of learned associations represented in a consciously accessible form. Cognitive-behavioural therapists, however, contend that conscious cognitions such as beliefs, plans and goals also influence behaviour and emotions.

With CBT, there seems to be some distinction between situationally accessed knowledge and verbally accessible knowledge. Cognitive theorists have argued that there are two cognitive systems that have different properties and different functions. One of these (situationally accessed knowledge) is automatic, out of conscious awareness, and involves large-scale information processing. Although we are consciously unaware of this kind of processing, we can become so when assessing thoughts and feelings. It can only be retrieved automatically when environmental input matches features of the stored memories. Therefore, when these aversive events are remembered, a person might become aware of the automatic activation of the emotions, thoughts, images and behavioural impulses. While the underlying representation remains inaccessible, its products become available to consciousness and permit a person to make inferences about the material stored in memory. Verbally accessible knowledge is a conscious process, which is slow and deliberate and acts on only a tiny fragment of the information available.

The techniques used by cognitive-behavioural therapists vary according to the problem identified. Clients differ in past experiences, the way in which any disorder manifests itself, the personal meaning they ascribe to their symptoms and the strategies they adopt to cope with the effects of the symptoms of the disorder. Some techniques are designed to change conscious beliefs, some teach skills in dealing with the difficulties encountered and others modify less accessible underlying structures in memory.

An example of a cognitive-behavioural strategy can be seen when therapists work with clients with specific phobias. Lang (1979) noted that representations underlying phobias contained three types of information.

- details of the location and physical characteristics of the feared situation (the stimulus elements)
- details of the verbal, physiological and behavioural responses that occurred in the situation (the response elements)
- an interpretation of the stimulus and response elements and of their significance for the individual (the meaning elements).

Once these three information representations have been detailed the therapist's role is to develop new memories within the client's perception that can be retrieved as situationally accessible knowledge. These memories are contrived to be as near to the original fear memory as possible, with the exception of the outcome. The client is encouraged to expose himself to the most realistic example of what he fears and to experience the same thoughts and feelings. The difference in therapy is that the experience is guided to allow the client to perfect the response to the fear memory and to master and become familiar with the fear rather than to avoid the stimulus. Clients exposed to their feared situations are therefore more likely to access this new memory containing fewer fearful response elements and a more benign meaning than they are to access the original memory.

When working with clients diagnosed as having one of the major psychiatric disorders, such as schizophrenia or depression, the underlying representations are thought to contain more abstract information. An example would be that a person with schizophrenia may have a number of social psychological and physical experiences that may be interwoven with each other such as social functioning issues, family relationships, illness beliefs, the effects of the illness, treatment beliefs, and views as to the course and prognosis of the illness, which will all impinge on his memory. The treatment of these disorders is generally of longer duration than the treatment of simple phobias and has a lower success rate.

CASE STUDY 4.1

Brenda is a 30-year-old woman who has been diagnosed as suffering from schizophrenia over the past 10 years. She is married with one child aged six. She is maintained in the community with support from the CPN service and depot medication. Approximately every two years she begins to hear voices of a persecutory nature and when this happens she normally has short-term admissions until the crisis is over. When being cared for in the community she is often unable to help around the house and frequently her husband has to do all the housework and look after their child. He is also quite supportive of her when she has problems though he has in the past lost his temper with her and there have been heated arguments. Her behaviour has also meant that they have few social support outlets, with other family members not wanting contact with Brenda or her husband.

In Brenda's case there are certain approaches that a nurse can take to alleviate the severity of the voices that she is experiencing. The therapist can start by elucidating issues relating to when the voices occur, how many voices there are, whether Brenda recognizes any voices, the severity of the voices, how long the voices last, what helps to ease the nature and severity of the voices and whether anything helps to stop the voices. From this the therapist can develop strategies for Brenda that can help alleviate and in time stop the voices. Examples of potential interventions are described by Barrowclough and Tarrier (1992).

The therapist may use attention switching where Brenda would be taught to concentrate on a positive or reinforcing image such as a beach holiday or a favourite family get-together when she experienced a delusion or hallucination. This is based on the notion that switching attention from one thought to another decreases the attention span and severity of the distracting delusion/hallucination. Another technique that may be used with Brenda is engaging in solitary activities when she starts to experience hallucination. This could include going for a walk alone or doing some exercise. The strategy is designed to provide some element of distraction while also reducing the amount of social arousal Brenda may be feeling on occasions.

FAMILY THERAPY

The development of family therapy began in the USA and UK in the 1950s. Much was based on the theories of Bateson *et al.* (1956) in relation to systems theory. Since then various schools of family therapy have been developed using the systemic approach as the starting point.

In family therapy, problems are viewed as parts of repetitive sequences of interaction which maintain and are maintained by the problem. Such sequences may be observed in the present or may be identified as recurring themes throughout the family history. These repetitive behavioural patterns and enduring beliefs are interconnected into what might be called a family system. Practitioners using a systemic approach aim to identify and change the meaning of a presenting problem within the context of such a system.

Systems theory

Basically, the theory states that the family is a system and should be considered as a whole and that its members and its characteristics can only be understood in terms of the total system. Each member influences and is influenced by the others: the whole is more than the sum of the parts. Once the family begins therapy, the therapist becomes part of the system.

In addition, all systems endeavour to maintain homeostasis. Homeostasis is described as the way in which families maintain a relatively constant way of functioning. In 'healthy' functioning families the group is able to develop in a way that allows both growth and security. However, when a family is dysfunctional it is unable to change or to develop naturally and gets stuck in repetitive ways of communicating and behaving.

The main theoretical concepts of systems theory are shown in Box 4.1.

Basic processes in family therapy

The major assertion is that the family is a rule-governed system; that is, its members behave among themselves in an organized repetitive manner and this pattern of behaviours can be abstracted as a governing principle of family life. The process of communication between family members is the main way in which therapists can observe and interpret how families organize their life.

There are three main family therapy schools:

- structural (Minuchin 1974, Minuchin and Fishman 1982)
- strategic (Haley 1976)
- Milan/systemic (Palazzoli *et al.* 1980).

Box 4.1   *Family systems theory*

- Families and other social groups are systems which are more than the sum of the properties of their parts.
- The operation of such systems is governed by certain general rules.
- Every system has a boundary, the properties of which are important in understanding how the system works.
- The boundaries are semipermeable; that is, some things can pass through them whereas other things cannot. In addition, some material can pass one way but not the other.
- Family systems tend to reach a relatively steady state. Growth and evolution are possible and indeed usual. Change can occur or be stimulated in many ways.
- Communication and feedback mechanisms between parts of a system are important in the functioning of the system.
- Events such as the behaviour of individuals in a family are best understood as examples of circular causality rather than as linear causality.
- Family systems, like other open systems, appear to have a purpose.
- Systems are made up of subsystems and themselves are parts of suprasystems.

Structural approach

This states that family structure is based on the invisible demands that organize the ways in which families work. There are repeated transactional patterns that underpin the system. The structure is defined by three main dimensions.

- *Boundary* – rules around which members participate or by which they are blocked from participation around a particular transaction.
- *Alignment* – between members (explicit or implicit). Who supports whom within the family and which family members oppose each other. In addition, is this support and conflict overt or covert?
- *Power* – the family member(s) whom other family members see as defining the agenda for the family. The appropriateness of the family member is also noted. An example would be if a young child, by virtue of their actions, was perceived as the person who governed what the family could or could not do.

The structural school has defined what it believes to be a well-functioning family system.

- The family can deal with stresses through flexibility.
- There are clearly marked boundaries.
- The power and the power hierarchy are clearly defined and the powerful

members of the family are appropriate for their age and role within the family.

The focus of the therapy is not the presenting problem, but the communication structure maintaining the problem. If there are difficulties, the therapeutic aim is to create a better family organization. This is achieved by the therapist joining the family in a leadership role and allowing the family to explore by:

- blocking dysfunctional transactions
- allowing the family to explore alternative responses.

A variety of techniques are utilized with the focus continuing to be on the transactional patterns of the family, the process rather than the content of communications.

The process of intervention uses the following methods.

- *Joining* – forming a therapeutic relationship with the family and allowing the therapist to observe the dysfunctional transactional patterns of the family.
- *Actualizing* – getting the family to enact a repetitive transaction and restructuring the way in which the transaction develops away from the normal repetitive communication and towards a new way of interaction. Two ways of doing this are to form boundaries around certain family members to allow them to develop a strategy that they were unable to do beforehand, and reframing, which has been defined by Watzlawick *et al.* (1974) as changing the conceptual and/or emotional setting or viewpoint in relation to which a situation is experienced and placing it in another frame which fits the 'facts' of the concrete situation equally well or even better and thereby changes its entire meaning.

Strategic theory

This is more of an ideology about the therapy, as opposed to a coherent school of treatment. It tries to look at what and who constitute the problem and how this can be brought into therapy. The problem is half of a cycle; the other half is what is engaged as a solution to a problem, i.e. the attempted solution. The process can be observed by the interview procedure adopted (Box 4.2).

Milan school approach

The underlying principle here is that change is not about knowing where the family should be, but evolving the family to where they should be.

The therapist conducts her investigation on the basis of feedback from the family in response to the information solicited about the relationship. This is usually through circular questioning whereby new questions are developed from the answers to the preceding questions. An example would be when a family member states whom within the family he would speak to if he were having personal problems, the next question may be addressed to another family member to ask whether they agreed with the statement. The rationale behind

---

Box 4.2   Interview procedure

1. Who has it?
2. How is it a problem?
3. What is the smallest change (step-by-step approach)?
4. What are the advantages and disadvantages of the change?

Prescription

1. Specific tasks set.
2. Behaviour to stay the same, but the situation is reframed. The principal technique utilized by the therapist is that of a 'one down position'. The therapist presents herself as a naive inquisitor with the family as expert witnesses about the family and the family system.

---

this is that the questioning challenges the family belief system which normally consists of all family members stating they agree with each other, without taking the side of any family member. It also allows the therapist to retain a neutral counselling position.

The therapist creates a hypothesis for the reasoning behind the problem. The hypothesis includes all parts of the family system with the behaviour of all the family members connected in a circular pattern with this behaviour connoted as good for the family. It is not the actual symptomatic behaviour that is connoted as positive. The family are normally given a paradoxical instruction that their behaviour is good for the family and that no change in the behaviour of the individual family members is good for the family system. The principles underlying this instruction are that the circular questioning will have already dynamically challenged the underlying beliefs of the family system which are seen as underpinning the dysfunctional communication patterns and that, with the therapist remaining neutral, the instruction allows the family system to gradually change at a rate with which the family feels comfortable.

If Brenda and her family were to be offered family therapy using the systems theory approach, the nurse would examine the underlying communication patterns between Brenda, her husband and her six-year-old child. Issues that might be examined would refer to the ways in which the family as a whole is hindered in developing. An example might be that when Brenda is talking her husband does not appear to listen or starts to pay attention to their child. If this happened on a consistent basis, the therapist would engage in some therapeutic intervention to stop this communication pattern from continuing. A structural approach would be to point out the behaviour to Brenda's husband and to encourage him to listen to Brenda's point of view. The underlying issue would be to try and ensure that both parents were treated fairly by each other and allowed each other to verbalize their thoughts and feelings in a safe and secure manner. Other types of family interaction may focus on specific problem areas such as trying to get Brenda and her husband to plan outings and to gradually get them to go out and socialize more. This would be a gradual process with constant monitoring from the therapist at each new stage.

SOCIAL THERAPY

Both Siegler and Osmond (1966) and Tyrer and Steinberg (1989) specified the existence of a social model that influenced the development and course of mental disorder. This social model regards the wider influence of social norms as more important than other influences as causes of mental illness. It has some similarities to the psychodynamic model in that the dynamic model sees the patient in the context of his personal relationships while the social model sees him as a player within society at large. However, there are specific differences which are shown in Box 4.3.

Box 4.3   Differences between the psychodynamic and social models

- *Psychodynamic model* – based on personal, highly specific information.
  Social model – based on general theories of groups, communities and cultures.
- *Psychodynamic model* – unconscious mental processes are important in causing mental illness.
  Social model – observed environmental factors explain mental illness.
- *Psychodynamic model* – past childhood conflicts explain present problems.
  Social model – current or recently experienced conflicts explain problems.
- *Psychodynamic model* – symptoms determined by symbolic significance.
  Social model – symptoms determined by nature or social events.
- *Psychodynamic model* – treated by group or personal psychotherapy.
  Social model – treated by social and environmental changes.

There have been a number of scientific advances in assessing social criteria, such as the Social Readjustment Rating Scale (Holmes and Rahe 1969) and the Social and Behavioural Disturbance Scale (Platt *et al.* 1980). To varying degrees life events have been shown to be important in the causation of mental illness. Cooper and Sylph (1973) suggest that negative events are seven times greater in patients with neurotic disorders. Negative life events have also been related to the onset of schizophrenic symptoms (Vaughn and Leff 1976, Zubin and Spring, 1977) and depression (Brown and Harris 1974). At times these social factors may not be apparent as they may be experienced months or even years before the onset of symptoms.

The social model maintains that mental illness is closely related to social factors. Therefore, unemployment, poor housing, living in deprived areas and poor occupational skills are all related to the likelihood of mental illness occurring. Because the social model sees the individual in the setting of society, it does not have set ideas of what constitutes psychiatric illness. The model is concerned that those who are diagnosed as being mentally ill will, once labelled, act the part. The roles of the nurse and client are determined by the norms of the society.

The social model sees the patient as a temporarily misplaced unit and so avoids labelling him as being ill. The aim of treatment is to help the individual to take up an acceptable role again rather than to correct a biochemical disturbance, exorcise an unresolved conflict or recondition behaviour. There are twin aims in the treatment model:

- to demonstrate to the patient that many of the fixed views that people hold about their condition are forced on them by society, for which they are not responsible
- to allow the patient to develop his own opinions and feelings free from social pressure.

This means that nurses should focus on treating the client in relation to problems such as independent living skills, social skills, unemployment, poverty and homelessness, as well as the stigma attached to having a mental illness.

Social skills training can be thought of as a series of learnt skills that are assessed and improved in certain ways. Trower et al. (1979) have developed a set of social skills exercises that can be applied with people who appear to be socially inadequate or have social deficits due to either institutionalization or the development of a severe mental disorder. One of the main areas of social skills training is assertiveness training which encourages direct but socially appropriate expressions of thoughts and feelings.

The most well-known treatment regime developed from social therapy theories is that of therapeutic communities. Therapeutic communities offer patients the ability to define their own social structure. The main principles of therapeutic communities were documented by Rappaport (1960) and are shown in Box 4.4.

Another way in which social therapy functions is by nurses and other health professionals trying to alter the way in which society deals with the mentally ill by changing social attitudes. Recent examples of psychiatric nurses being involved in this area include creating a women-only mental health house as an alternative to hospital admission (Cutting 1998) the promotion of mental health programmes for adolescents in schools (Puskar et al. 1997), carers roles as partners in dementia services (Simpson 1997) and awareness of educational and employment opportunities for people with mental health problems (Band et al. 1997).

In Brenda's case, interventions focusing on a social model approach would concentrate on developing skills as well as attempting to empower Brenda and to enable her to make decisions based on her own wishes and needs. The therapist

---

Box 4.4   The principles of the therapeutic community

- *Democracy* – all persons involved in the community, whether they be health professionals or staff, are equal. There is no hierarchy.
- *Openness* – all that occurs is open to all members of the community. Therefore there are no secrets.
- *Permissiveness* – there is an acceptance and toleration of behaviours and actions by all members of the community.
- *Reality confrontation* – where individuals or groups need to be confronted about their actions or behaviours, this is done by other members of the community, usually in group meetings. This encourages members of the community to take responsibility for the actions of everyone in the community.

---

could be involved in developing Brenda's practical skills, such as cooking and housework, or more vocational skills such as information technology training. The nurse could act as a facilitator in helping Brenda to gain work skills or even work experience. The aim of these interventions would be to develop or increase Brenda's skills in a variety of social situations which would lead to an increase in her self-esteem and self-worth. In addition, the therapist might start to encourage Brenda to develop assertiveness skills so that she could talk with her husband about her own thoughts and feelings in a confident and non-aggressive manner. This would again be advocated to improve her feelings of self-worth and help strengthen her relationship with her husband.

REFERENCES

Alligood, M.R. (1992) Empathy: the importance of recognising two types. *Journal of Psychosocial Nursing* 30(3): 14–17.

Authier, J. (1986) Showing warmth and empathy. In: Hargie, O. (ed.) *A Handbook of Communication Skills*. Croom Helm, London.

Baillie, L. (1996) A phenomenological study of the nature of empathy. *Journal of Advanced Nursing* 24: 1300–1308.

Barker, P. (1989) Rules of engagement. *Nursing Times* 85(51): 58–60.

Barrowclough, C. and Tarrier, N. (1992) *Families of Schizophrenic Patients: cognitive behavioural interventions*. Chapman and Hall, London.

Bateson, G., Jackson, D., Haley, J. and Weakland, J. (1956) Towards a theory of schizophrenia. *Behavioural Science* 1: 251–264.

Blacker, C.V. and Clare, A.W. (1987) Depressive disorder in primary care. *British Journal of Psychiatry* 150: 737–751.

Bond, G., Drake, R., Mueser, K. and Becker, D. (1997) An update on supported employment for people with severe mental illness. *Psychiatric Services* 48(3): 335–346.

Bradshaw, A. (1998) Charting some challenges in the art and science of nursing. *Lancet* 351(910): 438–440.

Brewin, C. (1996) Theoretical foundations of cognitive behaviour therapy for anxiety and depression. *Annual Review of Psychology* 47: 33–57.

Brown, G. and Harris, T. (1974) *The Social Origins of Depression*. Tavistock, London.

Brown, S.J. (1995) An interviewing style for nursing assessment. *Journal of Advanced Nursing* 21: 340–343.

Burnard, P. (1994) *Counselling Skills for Health Service Professionals*. Chapman and Hall, London.

Chinn, P. (1997) Response to 'The comforting interaction: developing a model of nurse–patient relationship'. *Scholarly Inquiry for Nursing Practice* 11(4): 345–347.

Clarkson, P. and Pokorny, M. (1994) *The Handbook of Psychotherapy*. Routledge, London.

Cooper, A. and Sylph, J. (1973) Life events and the onset of neurotic illness: an investigation in general practice. *Psychological Medicine* 3: 421–435.

Culley, S. (1992) Counselling skills: an integrative framework. In: Dryden, W. (ed.) *Integrative and Eclectic Therapy*. Open University Press, Milton Keynes.

Cutting, P. (1998) Clinical notice board. The women's services – providing an alternative to hospital admission. *Journal of Psychiatric and Mental Health Nursing* 5(3): 225–226.

Davidson, B. (1992) What can be the relevance of the psychiatric nurse to the life of a person who is mentally ill? *Journal of Clinical Nursing* 1: 199–205.

Egan, G. (1990) *The Skilled Helper*, 4th edn. Brooks Cole, Monterey.

Egan, G. (1994) *The Skilled Helper*, 5th edn. Brooks Cole, Monterey.

Fielding, R.G. and Llewelyn, S.P. (1987) Communication training in nursing may damage your health and enthusiasm: some warnings. *Journal of Advanced Nursing* 12(3): 281–290.

Gendlin, E. (1981) *Focusing*. Basic Books, New York.

Gould, D. (1990) Empathy: a review of the literature. *Journal of Advanced Nursing* 15(11): 1167–1174.

Gournay, K. (1995) Changing patterns in mental health care. *Psychiatric Care* 2(3): 93.

Gulland, A. (1998) Mental health crisis in the capital. *Nursing Times* 94(7): 19.

Haley, J. (1976). *Problem Solving Therapy*. Jossey Bass, San Francisco.

Heron, J. (1977) *Behavioural Analysis in Education and Training*. University of Surrey, Human Potential Resources Project.

Heyman, B. (1995) *Researching User Perspectives on Community Healthcare*, Chapman and Hall, London.

Hill, R.G., Hardy, P. and Shepherd, G. (1996) *Perspectives on Manic Depression: a survey of the Manic Depression Fellowship*. Sainsbury Centre for Mental Health, London.

Holmes, T. and Rahe, T. (1969) The Social Adjustment Rating Scale. *Journal of Psychosomatic Research* 19: 213–218.

Ivey, A. (1988) *Intentional Interviewing and Counselling*. Brooks Cole, Monterey.

Kahn, M.D. (1991) *Between the Therapist and the Client: the new relationship*. W.H. Freeman, New York.

Katayama, H. (1977) Role playing as a method to train nurses responsible for patient education: the most effective time to introduce role playing. *Japanese Journal of Health Psychology* 10(1): 1–11.

Lang, P. (1979) A bio-informational theory of emotional imagery. *Psychophysiology* 16: 495–512.

Lowenburg, J.S. (1994) The nurse patient relationship reconsidered: an expanded research agenda. *Scholarly Inquiry for Nursing Practice* 8(2): 167–184.

Masson, J. (1988) *Against Therapy*. Fontana, London.

McKay, M. (1983) *Messenger. The Communication Book.* New Harbinger, Oakland.

MIND (1992) *Stress on Women.* Policy paper on women and mental health. MIND, London.

Minuchin, S. (1974) *Families and Family Therapy.* Harvard University Press, Cambridge, Mass.

Minuchin, S. and Fishman, C. (1982) *Family Therapy Techniques.* Harvard University Press, Cambridge, Mass.

Morrison, P. and Burnard, P. (1991) *Caring and Communicating.* Macmillan, London.

Morrissey, M. (1998) A survey of information provision in mental health: what have we learned? *International Journal of Psychiatric Nursing.*

Morse, J.M. and Mitcham, C. (1997) Compathy: the contagion of physical distress. *Journal of Advanced Nursing* 26: 649–657.

Morse, J.M., Havens DeLuca, J.A. and Wilson, S. (1997) The comforting interaction: developing a model of nurse–patient relationship. *Scholarly Inquiry for Nursing Practice* 11(4): 321–343.

Murgatroyd, S. (1986) *Counselling and Caring.* Methuen, London.

Nelson-Jones, R. (1986) *Human Relationship Skills.* Cassell, London.

Palazzoli, M., Boscolo, L., Cecchin, G. and Prata, G. (1980) *Paradox and Counterparadox.* Aronson, New York.

Peplau, H. (1952) *Interpersonal Relations in Nursing.* Putnam, New York.

Pieranunzi, V.R. (1997) The lived experience of power and powerlessness in psychiatric nursing: a Heideggerian hermeneutical analysis. *Archives of Psychiatric Nursing* 11(3): 155–162.

Platt, S., Weyman, A., Hirsch, S. and Hewett, S. (1980) The Social Behaviour Assessment Schedule (SBAS): rationale, contents, scoring and reliability of a new interview schedule. *Social Psychiatry* 15: 43–55.

Puskar, K., Lamb, J. and Tusaei-Mumford, K. (1997) Teaching kids to cope: a preventive mental health nursing strategy for adolescents. *Journal of Child and Adolescent Psychiatric Nursing* 10(3): 18–28.

Rappaport, R. (1960) *Community as Doctor.* Tavistcok, London.

Rogers, C. (1961) *On Becoming a Person.* Houghton Mifflin, Boston.

Rogers, C. (ed.) (1967) *The Therapeutic Relationship and Its Impact.* University of Wisconsin Press, Madison.

Ryan, J. and Poster, E. (1989) The assaulted nurse: short-term and long-term responses. *Archives of Psychiatric Nursing* 3(6): 323–331.

Seligman, M.E. (1973) *Helplessness.* Freeman, New York.

Siegler, M. and Osmond, H. (1966) Models of madness. *British Journal of Psychiatry* 112: 1193–1203.

Simpson, R. (1997) Carers as equal partners in care planning. *Journal of Psychiatric and Mental Health Nursing* 4(5): 345–354.

Smail, D. (1978) *Psychotherapy: a personal approach.* Dent, London.

Stewart, W. (1983) *Counselling in Nursing: a problem-solving approach.* Harper and Row, London.

Trower, P., Bryant, B. and Argyle, M. (1979) *Social Skills and Mental Health.* Methuen, London.

Tyrer, P. and Steinberg, D. (1989) *Models for Mental Disorder: conceptual models in psychiatry.* John Wiley, Chichester.

Vaughn, C. and Leff, J. (1976) The influence of family and social factors in the course of mental illness. *British Journal of Psychiatry* 129: 125–137.

Watzlawick, P., Weakland, J. and Fisch, R. (1974) *Change: principles of problem formulation and problem resolution.* W.W. Norton, New York.

Zderad, L. (1969) Empathic nursing: realisation of a human capacity. *Nursing Clinics of North America* **4**(4): 655–662.

Zubin, J. and Spring, B. (1977) Vulnerability: a new view of schizophrenia. *Journal of Abnormal Psychology* **86**: 103–126.

5 THE NURSE AS REFLECTOR

Sheila Forster and Andrew Thomas

OBJECTIVES

After reading this chapter, you should be able to:

- understand the importance of knowing yourself as a powerful tool in the use of reflection
- describe the key models of self which underpin self-awareness
- give an account of the components of the self and the factors that influence its development
- understand the models of reflection which aid self-awareness and its growth
- look at your own practice in the light of various methods of reflection and apply the appropriate one(s) to your clinical area.

INTRODUCTION

It is often said that the most important thing that people bring to nursing is not theoretical knowledge or technical skills (although these are, of course, very important), it is themselves: their basic character and personality. If one accepts this viewpoint, can an argument be made that training and education are unnecessary in nursing in anything other than the so-called 'pure' sciences, i.e. biological science?

It is hardly likely that this argument would be supported by many (if any) nurses today. However, as pointed out in Chapter 1, communication skills and therapeutic use of self were only made explicit in the 1982 syllabus of training for psychiatric nurses.

Therefore, for many years psychiatric nurses managed to survive with barely any formal education in this area. The impact of this state of affairs on the quality of care offered and the effects on mental health nursing as a profession to some extent remain with us today despite great efforts to address this shortcoming.

This chapter supports the work previously carried out to promote the central importance of self-awareness and the essential activity of reflection for the mental health nurse, so that quality of care and the professionalism of mental health nursing can continue to increase.

Nursing can only progress and fully achieve professional status, as defined by Allan and Jolley (1987), if each nurse takes responsibility for her own development of self-awareness and reflective ability. Since the act of nursing is primarily a team activity, individual progress can and should be shared, thus ensuring that the individuals within the team, the team itself and, ultimately, the body of nursing will benefit. This bottom-up approach should improve the outcome for the consumers of the service – the patients/clients – and result in care of the highest standard.

So, what are the responsibilities of individual mental health nurses? In a nutshell, the willingness and increasing ability to consider and explore how they affect the world around them; how that world affects them; why this is so; and what they are able and willing to do about it. By actively seeking answers to these questions in relation to their practice, nurses will find that they respond to clients/patients more individually; current practices will be challenged, evaluated and, consequently, improved upon; knowledge will be increased; professional effectiveness will be enhanced; and increased professional growth will take place.

If each nurse rises to the above challenge, the wisdom of Benner's (1984) assertion that theory is embedded in practice will be recognized and her observation that there is a barrier between nursing as it ought to be and nursing as it is, with teachers advocating the former and nurses knowing the latter, will no longer be valid.

To meet this challenge, certain qualities are required. Dewey (1933) identified the main ones as being: having an open mind; being responsible; having a whole-hearted approach in order to consider all sides of an argument; being able to consider the outcomes of actions you might wish to undertake; and taking active control over your own education and practice. Therefore, to assess the presence or absence of these qualities, some degree of self-exploration (heightened self-awareness) is a prerequisite to the activity of reflecting in or on action.

THE IMPORTANCE OF SELF-AWARENESS

The concept of self

In earlier chapters, the centrality of interpersonal relationships in mental health nursing has been firmly established. The widely held view (e.g. Peplau 1991, Sullivan, 1953) that interpersonal relationships underpin all nursing practice warrants an exploration of the implications for, and the responsibilities of, nurses if they are to promote what Travelbee (1971) refers to as 'therapeutic use of self'.

The concept of self has occupied psychologists, philosophers and theologians for many years. This has led to numerous theories emerging, for example those of Allport (1961), Erikson (1963), Freud (1961), Mead (1934) and Sullivan (1953) – the only common thread appearing to be that the concept of self is complex!

Whilst it is acknowledged that all these theories can inform mental health nursing, Burnard (1985) maintains that the existential school of philosophy, particularly the work of Sartre (1956), and the psychoanalytical school, notably Jung (1978), have been the most illuminating. Put simply, Sartre's work focused on the concept of authenticity, the importance of acting as honestly and genuinely as possible, whereas Jung took a transpersonal viewpoint which acknowledges that we do not exist in isolation from one another and therefore, our concept of self will be influenced by, and will influence, others; an important factor to be borne in mind when reflecting in and on practice.

Taking Sartre's work as a basis and acknowledging the contribution made by Jung, Laing (1959) proposed that the self can be 'true' and 'false', the true self being the inner, private self, and the false self being that shown to others, i.e., responding to the expectations/needs of others and in so doing, being artificial and insincere. Recognizing the importance of this work and its implications for the role of the mental health nurse, Burnard (1985) developed two models of self to assist nurses to explore the concept in relation to their personal and professional roles and, as a consequence, enhance their level of self-awareness.

The first of these models Burnard calls 'a simple model of self'. This comprises three overlapping circles of equal size. Each circle represents one aspect (or domain) of self, namely thoughts, feelings and behaviour. Burnard explains these terms as follows.

> By thoughts is meant the process of ideas, puzzlement, problem-solving that makes up our mental life. By feelings is meant the emotional aspects of our being: happiness, grief, love, anger, etc. Behaviour refers to any action that we carry out and also to the spoken word and to what is usually referred to as non-verbal behaviour: eye contact, facial expression, gestures, proximity to others, etc. (Burnard 1985, p. 4)

The overlapping of these domains reminds us that whatever happens in one domain will affect the other two, thinking is always accompanied by feelings and behaviour, all behaviours produce thought and feelings, all feelings lead to or arise out of behaviours and thoughts.

Despite the simplicity of this model, the implications for nursing practice are wide ranging. Burnard's second model (1985) is more complex and, as such, enables these implications to be focused upon more explicitly. The influence of both Laing (1959) and Jung (1978) is apparent in this framework, which Burnard has called 'a comprehensive model of self'. This model proposes the existence of inner and outer aspects of self (based on Laing's real and false selves). The outer self is what we present to those around us and Burnard maintains that this is exclusively the domain of behaviour. To support this claim he makes the point that the only way we can convey our thoughts and feelings to others is through the behaviours we display. (If this is accepted, does this indicate that at any one time we are only effectively communicating with and responding to one third of the other person's self? Another important point to reflect on!)

The inner self relates to the private aspect, what goes on in our heads and bodies. This incorporates the four aspects of human experience identified by

Jung: thinking (all aspects, logical and illogical, of our mental processes), feeling (the emotional aspects of the person), sensing (use of the special senses, i.e. touch, taste, smell, hearing and sight to gain information) and intuiting (insights and knowledge gained independently of the senses).

The employment of models of self such as these can, and does, lead to a greater understanding of the complex concept of self. Recognizing and appreciating the impact we have on the world and how we react/respond to what the world throws at us will be beneficial to our personal and professional growth; in other words, our level of self-awareness will increase.

Self-awareness

Developing self-awareness is an intentional act, it does not just happen. Discipline, perseverance and consistency are required so that aspects of self (behavioural, psychological or physical) are noted and examined continually. As stated earlier, the concept of self is complex. It is shaped by many factors which impact on who we are. Whilst a psychoanalytical exploration is not being promoted here, some consideration needs to be given to our developmental years and the effect that these have on us.

Developmental theories abound, for example (1969) and Sullivan (1953), and these can help us to recognize, appreciate and explore the attitudes, beliefs and values systems we have adopted and developed, for it is these that determine not only how we see ourselves but how we see and respond to others. Argyle (1983) asserts that the following points reflect this and influence the development of our self:

- the reaction of other people to us
- comparing ourselves with others
- the past, present and future roles that we play
- identification of models.

Pause for a moment and think of the frequency with which you use the term 'self'. Now look at the context in which this word can be used. It is likely that you have covered a wide range of applications such as 'self-interest', 'self-indulgent;, 'self-image', 'self-esteem', 'self-disclosure' 'self-concept', 'self-conscious'. Each of these terms has some bearing on the self and the way in which they are used, about yourself or others, can be an indicator of your level of self-awareness.

Oliver (1993) suggests that the three most important terms to consider in relation to exploring/enhancing self-awareness are 'self-image', 'ideal self' and 'self-esteem'.

Self-image

Self-image, as the name implies, refers to the way we see ourselves. To gain an understanding of another's self-image, it is helpful to ask them to describe themselves. Before reading on, do just that – briefly jot down a description of yourself. When we carry out this type of activity the outcome is often dominated by physical attributes (body image). Was yours?

The description given will invariably be value laden, not always positive and less than objective; what is more, it may not equate to others' perception of you! For example, an individual might see and describe themselves physically as being built like a beanpole, with greying hair and a nose that is too prominent. Others may perceive this person as a tall, slim, elegant, distinguished individual who has classic Roman features! It follows that our body image will affect other facets of our self-image and the picture that emerges may be less than flattering because what we think we are conflicts with what we would prefer to be, i.e. the ideal self.

Ideal self

The need to examine the self-image against the ideal self and recognize the differences is very important for mental health nurses, not only to enhance their own self-awareness but so that they can understand their clients/patients better. Many of the problems seen in mental health settings are due to conflicts arising from the individual's inability to live up to their ideal self which, as a consequence, has an adverse effect on their self-esteem.

Self-esteem

Oliver (1993) maintains that self-esteem develops out of our self-image and, as such, it is a product of how others respond to us based on what we contribute, or fail to contribute, to society. Fundamentally, our level of self-esteem is a personal evaluation of our self-image and its relationship with the ideal self. Because of the subjective nature of this measurement and the fact that self-esteem will vary to some extent over time and in response to changing societal expectations/environmental circumstances, it is essential to regularly revisit the following questions.

- How do I affect the world around me?
- How does the world affect me?
- Why is this so?
- What am I able/willing to do about it?

If we can follow Sartre's lead by responding to these questions honestly and genuinely and be willing to take on Burnard's suggestion of exploring the inner and outer aspects of self then self-awareness will be increased and we will be better placed to reflect on our professional practice more effectively.

THE NURSE AS REFLECTOR

Darbyshire (1993) stated that nursing 'is more fashion conscious than a catwalk full of supermodels' (p. 26) and certainly increasing amounts of published material have demonstrated the value of reflection to nursing practice during the past few years (Palmer *et al.* 1994, Rolfe 1997, Schon 1991). It will be argued here that unless the idea of reflection is fully understood and implemented, it will become the latest 'fashion icon' and will be discarded. Although there have been criticisms of it as a tool, this chapter will demonstrate that in the context of mental health nursing, which we see as a highly creative and individual process, the use of reflection, when applied wholeheartedly, is invaluable and should be encouraged. Minghella and Benson (1995) argue strongly that reflection plays a vital part in the understanding of the interactive, interpersonal relationships that are at the heart of mental health nursing.

Having looked at the importance to the process of reflection of self-awareness on the part of the nurse, we will now look more closely at these models and the nature of reflection so that its value in nursing practice can be demonstrated. In spite of growing emphasis in the literature, reflective methods for use in clinical practice have also been criticized. While Jarvis (1992), for example, argues that there is a danger of habituation when carrying out nursing tasks and that therefore the use of reflection provides continual new learning situations, Greenwood (1993), on the other hand, believes that it is overused and relies too heavily on subjective interpretation after the event has passed. If reflective processes are to be used, writers such as Jarvis (1992) and Johns (1996) encourage the use of a model that is both structured and asks pertinent rather than vague questions.

Why reflect?

The value of using reflective methods has been addressed by many writers. Benner (1984) makes it very clear that without the constant use of reflection, new knowledge will not be discovered.

> *A wealth of untapped knowledge is embedded in the practices and the 'know-how' of expert nurse clinicians, but this knowledge will not expand or fully develop unless nurses systematically record what they learn from their own experience. (p. 11)*

It is precisely this 'untapped knowledge' that the process of reflection can uncover when it is done in a systematic way. Schon (1995) points out that a crisis of confidence in the professions is happening, caused by scepticism about the delivery of competent services. Reflection is one method of 'prodding' in order to ask the question: 'Is what I am doing in the best interests of the patient and can I justify why I am doing it?'. In mental health nursing particularly, the use of nursing models is often seen as having little value since they encourage the stereotyping of the patient and often result in fitting the patient to the model (Johns 1996) whereas the reverse should apply if we accept that each encounter with each patient has to rely on an individual approach. It is surely only by applying the principles of reflection that we can do this, without relying on care models with their accompanying drawbacks.

Possibly one reason for resistance to using a reflecting method is that it is more time consuming than employing a more traditional approach. However, when asking mental health nurses which model they base their care on, it is common to get the wry response accompanied by matching non-verbal behaviour, 'the eclectic one'. It would appear from this that many mental health nurses are more comfortable basing their clinical care on the results of active observation and reflection rather than on a more rigid adherence to one nursing model.

However, simply justifying the use of reflection on a single ground is not adequate. There are several reasons for using this method (Palmer *et al.* 1994). One main factor which ties in with Schon (1995) is that it improves and evaluates practice more thoroughly, since the practitioner is continually questioning why and how something worked or the reasons for failure in the situation. Street (1991) feels that many nurses rely heavily on 'instinct', which may be born out of years of experience, and that reflection can identify more clearly the components of the action being taken, which then leads to greater professional growth and a more creative approach to the patient. This is empha-sized by Emden (1991) who links reflective practice with the mature nurse who has a strong commitment to continually improving standards of clinical practice to the benefit of the client.

Durgahee (1996) believes that the effects of learning by reflection are to augment one's critical thinking, to enhance listening and observational skills and to gain increased insight into clinical situations. This increase in critical thinking will lead in turn to greater confidence and assertiveness, which is perhaps most appropriate to the recently qualified mental health nurse who may feel lacking in clinical experience. Critical thinking is defined by Brookfield (1987) as having four components:

- identifying and challenging the assumptions that are frequently made in the workplace about practice and those with whom we work
- appreciating the importance to critical thinking of the context in which we work
- having the imagination to explore alternatives to decisions and actions
- continually questioning the care given to patients with a healthy scepticism.

Summary
We reflect in order to:

- respond to clients in an individual way
- challenge and evaluate current practices
- enhance our knowledge in a dynamic fashion
- grow professionally
- increase our professional effectiveness.

If, therefore, the aim of mental health nursing is to enter into a dynamic, creative relationship with clients, rather than a series of 'tasks', then mental health nurses must continually question their interactions and the impact of those interactions. Reflective practice seems to answer that challenge but to be systematic, we must also understand the basis for learning from reflection.

Learning and reflection

Benner (1984) has provided us with the basis for looking at learning through experience. She considers the gradual growth of expertise through exposure to clinical situations which demand a degree of decision making proportionate to the nurse's experience, beginning at novice stage and culminating at the level of expert.

As a novice, one's behaviour is governed by rules, which means that behaviour at first tends to be inflexible and cautious due to a lack of confidence. At this stage, the novice may well be watching the more experienced nurse with some degree of questioning, since behaviour may be seen which does not 'go by the book'. By the stage of expert, the nurse can see the situation as a whole rather than as a set of factors which are considered separately. Continuing use of reflection on practice has here given rise to an intuitive grasp of what is happening.

At the novice stage, the nurse may see the expert as performing multifaceted tasks effortlessly, whereas what is really happening is a continuous process of assimilation, where the nurse is combining stimuli from many sources: the client, other professionals, the environment and knowledge from past experiences (Rolfe 1997). Psychologists call this process 'chunking', where cognitive or behavioural units are put together so that they are seen holistically as a total unit. At first seen as isolated cases, the expert nurse is able, with the use of intuition born from experience, to put them into a 'slot'. This does not imply the formation of stereotypes but rather the experience of a certain familiarity with a situation. Kolb (1984) sees this as a four-stage process (the learning cycle) moving from the experience as seen in practice to observation and reflection, to generalization and conceptualization which in turn leads to active experimentation – one of the main aims of the reflective process.

CASE STUDY 5.1

Tim, a 36-year-old male, suffering from a severe mental health problem, is demanding to leave the ward unescorted. His non-verbal behaviour is threatening and his speech content is delusional and hostile.

THE NOVICE NURSE

At this stage, the nurse lacks experience and, although aware of what should be done, has a problem choosing the correct nursing intervention from those that she has available. She knows the 'textbook' approach but lacks clinical familiarity with its implementation and may not feel completely convinced that her selected way of managing this potentially violent situation is the right one.

This hesitancy may be apparent to both other colleagues and the patient, who may take advantage of it in order to intimidate the nurse further. The nurse may respond by relying on the policy and procedure manual, considering utilizing the nurse's holding power under the Mental Health Act 1983 (an extreme reaction) rather than asking the client to express his feelings in a more quiet environment and giving him the time to talk through what his real needs are.

At present, the novice nurse is feeling intimidated by Tim and reacting on a basic level to that intimidation, which is not helpful either to her confidence or to Tim and the other patients.

THE NURSE AS EXPERT

On the other hand, the expert nurse has a wealth of experience to draw on and uses his knowledge of the client and his nursing skills to maximum effect. He intuitively knows what interventions to use and in which order. He is aware of his own feelings and reacts to this situation by using the model of nursing he either practices or feels is right for the situation.

His skills are honed to his practice. He will realize the potential dangers in this situation and attempt to diffuse the situation by being non-confrontational yet firm; for example, asking Tim if he would like to sit down and talk about what is bothering him, knowing that allowing Tim to ventilate his feelings and offering support to him will help him to become less hostile. He will be aware of the non-verbal messages that he is transmitting to Tim at the same time, demonstrating that he is not hostile or panicked by his behaviour and using his communication skills to increase his rapport with Tim. He will have a feeling of what Tim is reacting to and how he may react in the next few minutes and will have made physical and mental preparations for all eventualities such as alerting staff to be near at hand to reassure other clients on the ward and to be ready to step in should it be necessary.

At this stage of practice, he is completely aware of how he feels and has complete faith in his practice. He shows none of the hesitancy that the novice shows and uses his relationship with Tim to enable Tim to trust him and interact more effectively with his immediate environment.

Darbyshire (1993) feels that in nursing recently there has been a shift away from what Schon (1974) termed 'technical rationality', which is learning influenced by objectivity and detached analysis, towards what Dreyfus and Dreyfus (1985) called 'deliberative rationality'. In this type of learning, the nurse becomes more flexible, the use of flexibility is encouraged and a more contemplative approach to care is adopted. This can be clearly seen in many mental health areas where task is less important than process but it relies heavily on nurses using perception combined with reflection and then being prepared to 'strike out' if necessary into new methods of solving a problem or working with a client, at the risk of not being understood by one's peers.

Similarly, Van Manen (1991) describes four types of learning through reflection which the nurse can employ in different situations. First is knowledge gained through anticipatory reflection, where a lot of preparatory work can be done before the situation occurs, i.e. gaining information, preparing the environment according to a perceived need, etc. Second, he describes the use of active reflection in action, being aware of what is going on around you and working within it. Darbyshire (1993) points out that this is the area of reflective practice that causes most problems in a nursing context. This could be because of time pressures or more simply because it is difficult to mentally 'stand back' at the same time as carrying out a nursing intervention. This will be covered in the last section of this chapter. The third area is 'mindfulness', which means being involved consciously and immediately in a situation that can be 'unpacked' later, either individually or as part of a team process as described by Graham (1995). This is perhaps particularly valuable as a learning process that can take place during the shift handover period. The final type of recollective, where after the event the nurse can analyse what happened and why it was successful or not. However, this relies on accurate mental or written recording of the intervention.

The basis of nursing knowledge

The work of Carper (1978) is an attempt to demonstrate the different types of knowledge that the nurse can draw on to increase skills and influence nursing practice and it is interesting for nurses to look critically at how and why these are used in their nursing practice and where there are weak areas or blind sports. The four types of knowledge are described as follows.

Empiric

This is seen as the testing and observation of theories to provide scientific evidence of the importance of a process. Since the introduction of Project 2000, there has been great emphasis on this, as nurse education increasingly establishes a sound research-based body of knowledge on which the student nurse can draw. It also includes knowledge gained from other disciplines from which, after reflection, the nurse gains perspectives which are unique to the individual's own area of nursing practice. Although this type of knowledge is seen as the basis for sound nursing practice, Carper (1978) recognized that other types of knowledge also need to influence nursing practice, since using skills and practices based only on empirical knowledge would result in a very inflexible approach, which is still evident in a minority of nurses who feel uncomfortable using other types of knowledge (the 'We've always done it this way' approach).

Ethics

This is the judgement-making approach to any clinical situation. It is important when using this angle that nurses reflect on their own values and, through this reflection and discussion with others, that they become more aware of the basis for their decisions, as objective and born out of personal beliefs rather than a subjective 'knee jerk' reaction.

Aesthetics

Schon (1987) saw this as the art of nursing, combining the use of intuition with experience to provide answers to an unexpected situation. There is the danger of losing objectivity here, and relying too heavily on personal intuition, which takes us on to the importance of regular reflection and debate on what is actually being achieved in any nursing situation.

Personal

This emphasizes the centrality of self-awareness, since unless you know yourself you cannot be aware of why you are acting in certain ways and such actions then become meaningless. For example, it is very difficult to help a patient who is suffering severe depression without having an understanding of how we ourselves could be vulnerable to emotional pain and distress and in turn, how that would affect us.

> *In using personal knowledge, a new perspective comes into play as the individual perceives him or herself to be able to adjust or modify a response, recognizing the personal aspect of the situation which is context bound in the here and now. (Robinson and Vaughan 1992, p. 10)*

The process of reflection

Reflection is seen as being initiated by some unease in a clinical situation:

> *There is some puzzling, or troubling or interesting phenomenon with which the individual is trying to deal. As he tries to make sense of it, he also reflects on the understandings which have been implicit in his action, understandings which he surfaces, criticizes, restructures, and embodies in further action. (Schon 1995, p. 50)*

Learning in this context is associated with 'thinking on your feet' and Schon (1995) differentiates between reflection-on-action, where the situation is analysed after it has happened to discover the knowledge that was used in the situation and whether it could have been handled differently, and reflection-in-action, where the nurse gains a perception of something new about the situation, while engaged in practice. In the second type of reflection, a three-stage process emerges. First, rather than attempting to place the practice problem in a framework of similar situations that have been encountered before, the nurse approaches the problem as though it is unique and has not occurred before. Second, the features particular to the situation are discovered: this becomes a gradual process with more features being discovered, so that the situation can then be reframed. Lastly, the nurse performs 'artistically'; to a novice this may seem to be simple and spontaneous but in reality it is the result of a complex set of interwoven responses.

> *Even with very simple tasks such as wound dressing, the difference is striking: the expert nurse would perform the required actions swiftly and deftly and without conscious thought, whereas the reflective practitioner would think about every move, every decision, relating them to this patient in this situation. (Rolfe 1997, p. 96)*

Reflection makes caring visible, enabling it to be acknowledged, affirmed, valued. The necessary commitment can be nurtured, self knowing realized, aesthetic skills honed to respond appropriately, and the environment of care challenged. (Johns 1996)

The value of reflection has been clearly demonstrated from many sources and yet many nurses resist its use in the clinical context. This may simply be due to a lack of information about different methods that can be used in different scenarios, which the following section will address, but also because it is still a relatively new approach which, being unfamiliar, also causes anxieties.

Methods of reflection

The final section of this chapter will explore the various methods that can be used to reflect critically on nursing practice, which range widely from informal to formal and individual to group methods. It is important to emphasize that the context of where the nursing care is taking place may influence the type of reflection that is undertaken.

Types of reflective methods range widely from formal to informal, written to verbal and structured to more loosely structured but they all have in common the desire to create new knowledge and insight into practice. Lumby (1981) points out that 'the explosion of texts addressing reflection and reflective practice perhaps best illustrates a frustration with traditional methods of inquiry' (p. 93) and Johns (1996) states that traditional models of nursing do not encourage the use of reflection but set the trap of matching the patient to the model which can result in a return to task-orientated nursing. Regularly using a method of reflection with which you are comfortable, helps to ensure that the client with whom you are working or the activity in which you are involved comes under closer scrutiny and is not seen merely as a routine process.

The reflective journal

At the novice stage the reflective journal is often simplistic and relies heavily on the narrative, as demonstrated by the following example, written by a student nurse reflecting two months into the course on his experience of the selection interview.

When I arrived I noticed that some people were a lot better dressed than me, and I was annoyed that I had not thought more about presenting myself in a better light. This in turn meant that I was put off and did not respond well at first in the interview. ... I was last on the interview list and had to sit in the corridor for over an hour and no one had told us where to go for a drink, so I was also feeling quite annoyed. ... All in all I didn't feel that I was presenting myself at my best. Looking back, the experience taught me a lot about being better prepared and needing to be more assertive.

As it stands, this excerpt (although small) shows that the student is self-aware and is able to start to analyse what an experience meant. Consider, however, the following excerpt from a student who was a year into the course, talking about a period of disorganization in providing teachers for mental health sessions.

> *I was looking forward to the introduction to mental health nursing as this is the branch that I am most interested in. For the first lecture nobody arrived to teach us and after a good half hour someone was found to stand in for the missing lecturer and he talked to us in rather a haphazard way about one or two aspects of mental health nursing. A similar thing happened for the next two lectures; someone who was unprepared ended up standing in to take the session.*
>
> *During these three lectures I felt embarrassed for the staff who were placed in difficult situations, but also very disappointed that I had learnt so little about an area that is probably going to be profoundly important in my life. I felt that it was important to let the lecturers know that I was not angry with them personally for the breakdown in the system and I spoke out to that effect. If similar circumstances arise again, I think the group rep should make a point of seeing the subject leader and asking for the lost time to be made up and I regret that we didn't do this then as I feel I have missed out.*

Both these excerpts from reflective diaries are fairly unstructured and, although useful to the student for expressing feelings, would benefit from a more structured approach so that each angle of the experience can be analysed more methodically. For example, the description of the event can be separated from the reflection, as shown below.

Event	Reflection
Mrs Jones was sitting on the side of her bed and didn't look well. She suddenly collapsed and started to hyperventilate.	I felt very scared because I had never seen anyone do that before, and I didn't know what to do.

Having here identified that the problem is caused by lack of knowledge on the part of the student, either she or her mentor can then look at what learning or teaching may be appropriate.

Another method of trying to pin down what is being reflected upon is more structured still. Johns (1996) looks at the use of the Burford model to boost standards of care, which entails asking the following questions.

- *Core question* – what information do I need in order to nurse this person/family?
- *Cue questions:*
  - Who is this person?
  - What health event brings this person into a hospital or health environment?
  - How is this person feeling?
  - How has this event affected this person's usual life patterns and rules?
  - How do I feel about this person?
  - How can I help this person?

– What is important for this person to make his/her stay in hospital comfortable?
– What support does this person have in life?
– How does this person view the future for him/herself and others?

As has already been stated, it is important that the structure used, whether complex or simple, is comfortable to users and they should be encouraged to find a method that suits their working style.

Consider another method used by a student in rostered service, reflecting on a violent incident. The questions she asked were as follows.

- What did I do? (I was initially frightened and then I watched what X (my mentor) was doing and went along with that.)
- What did the client do? (Because X did not get too close and kept her voice calm, the client started to slow his behaviour down, although he still looked very angry.)
- What did the others in the team do? (X was dealing with it really but there were to other nurses on the ward and one was staying close to the other clients and the other was fairly close to the client in case he became aggressive again.)
- What was the outcome? (X managed to persuade the client to move away from the chair that he had been holding on to and into the smoking room, where she accompanied him with the other nurse).
- What did I learn from this experience. (My main thoughts are that I need to be aware more of my own non-verbal responses. I noticed that X kept her hands by her sides and looked very relaxed, so that the client picked this up, and that her voice stayed calm. I felt quite unsure of how to get the client to calm down and I think that if I had been alone in this situation, I would have showed the client that I was scared which wouldn't have made things any better.)

Practice write-ups

These were introduced by Gormley (1997) as an instrument that attempts to remedy the theory–practice gap that has been widely written about (Alexander 1982). Practice write-ups 'encourage students to analyse routine experiences of nursing practice and utilize them as learning situations' (Gormley 1997, p. 54).

He describes the process as having three stages. The first is the consideration of the core skill being used in a particular situation by the use of guided reading, clinical observation and clinical practice. Secondly, under supervision, the student analyses key features of the experience in order finally to produce a fresh approach to the situation.

CRITICAL INCIDENT TECHNIQUE

This technique or set of procedures derives from ethnology, the study of animal behaviour. Until Flanagan (1954) formalized this technique, it had been used, albeit in a piecemeal fashion, to identify effective and ineffective performance in human beings in a wide range of activities.

Since Flanagan focused and refined this technique, which he described as being appropriate to:

> ... *any observable human activity that is sufficiently complete in itself to permit inferences and predictions to be made about the person performing the act ... an incident must occur in a situation where the purpose or intent of the act seems fairly clear to the observer and where its consequences are sufficiently definite to leave little doubt concerning its effects. (Flanagan 1954, p. 327)*

it has been employed as a research methodology in nursing to investigate aspects of practice (Crow 1978, Cunningham 1979, Long 1976, Sims 1976). Cormack (1983) used the critical incident technique in an attempt to describe psychiatric nursing. In his rationale for using this method, Cormack cites Clamp's (1980) description of critical incidents:

> ... *snapshot views of the daily work of the nurse ... the advantages of this technique are that they provide a sharply focused description in which opinions, generalizations and personal judgements are reduced to a minimum. (Cormack 1983, p. 31)*

Accepting the above, what is being promoted here is that individual nurses should be researchers into their own practice. The question that arises, in light of Clamp's description, is how feasible it is to objectively observe, record, analyse and draw inferences from one's own behaviour and the situations in which one practises.

In the following section the component parts of critical incident technique will be explored, suggestions as to employing the technique will be made and an example of its effective use will be presented. The outcome should leave little doubt that the answer to the above question is in the affirmative and that critical incident technique is a worthy and rewarding method of reflection.

Examples of situations which lend themselves to exploration using the critical incident technique are:

- any personal action taken which made an impact on a patient's care provision
- events that went particularly well
- events that did not go according to plan
- situations which capture and exemplify the essence of mental health nursing
- personally or professionally demanding situations
- circumstances from which it was felt significant learning took place.

To record critical incidents, the following format is suggested.

- Write a detailed description of the event – where and when it happened, your own and others' involvement/actions.

- Identify what it was about the event that made it significant for you and record how you felt at the time.
- Identify and explain the most satisfactory and least satisfactory aspects of the situation. Based on the outcomes of this activity, consider what you might have done differently.
- Consider what action, if any, you will take as a result of this reflection and record the reasons for your choice(s).

CASE STUDY 5.2

A situation arose on an acute admission unit which involved John, a mental health branch nursing student, who, shortly after the event, was advised by his supervising staff nurse to subject it to critical incident analysis. John wrote as follows:

Toward the end of an early shift, and just after the consultant psychiatrist's case conference, I was instructed by Mary, the staff nurse, to tell Mike, a patient, that he would not now be allowed home for the weekend because his medication had been altered and he would need to be observed on the ward for the next few days.

I approached Mike in the lounge area of the ward and asked if I could have a word. He said 'I don't feel much like talking at the moment, is it important?'. I started to explain that it was about his planned temporary leave but before I could finish Mike became angry and abusive. I tried to calm him down but it seemed to make matters worse. He then strode off towards the dormitory, pushing over a chair as he went and shouting that 'No jumped-up little jobsworth' would tell him what to do and 'If I want to go home, I f—ing well will – you try and stop me'.

I was shocked at his reaction, particularly since I had not been able to deliver the whole message. I was also a bit annoyed that he felt he had to insult me as I thought we had a good relationship up until this happened. Even though I felt a bit apprehensive, I decided to follow Mike to make sure he was okay. When I asked him if he was all right he told me, in a loud voice, 'No, now f— off and leave me alone'. By now I was starting to feel anxious and unsure of how best to deal with the situation but also felt I needed to stand my ground so I told him that whilst I understood his disappointment I didn't think it was helpful for him to get so angry and be so rude. Mike responded to this by telling me to get out of his sight before he did something he might regret. At this point Mary, having heard the raised voices, appeared and advised me to go to the ward office to prepare for the shift handover and to tell the ward manager where she was and who she was with. Despite feeling like a naughty school boy who had just been told off, I did as she said. Mary joined me some 10 minutes later having effectively defused the situation with Mike.

My initial reaction when asked to explore this incident was annoyance. I felt I had been set up to fail. I had done as I was told, acted in good faith and ended up being insulted and threatened for my trouble. However, having calmed down and explored the incident more objectively, a number of important points came to light.

First, I agreed to give Mike a message without thinking through the possible consequences of this; I should have considered how this news might have been received and reacted to by Mike rather than trying to impress Mary by dutifully following her instructions. Having approached Mike I should have questioned whether the ward lounge was the most appropriate environment in which to convey this information. Rather than insisting on trying to give the message, I should have acknowledged Mike's initial response and invited him to elaborate why he didn't feel like talking at that moment. (It transpired that Mike was aware that his leave would be cancelled from his discussion with the consultant earlier in the morning; unfortunately, Mary had not been party to this. Mike later confirmed that he felt his 'nose was being rubbed in it' by being asked to discuss the matter again so soon after receiving the bad news.)

Looking back, I now realize that I responded to Mike's aggression and insults more on a personal level than a professional one. My need to stand my ground was an attempt to assert my authority. This, consequently, led to a will struggle developing between Mike and myself which reduced my ability to appreciate and understand Mike's situation. I'm not surprised Mike appeared to resent it when I told him I did understand (because it must have been obvious that I did not!)

Even though this incident has served to highlight a number of shortcomings on my part, I feel that, having explored it, this has been a very good, albeit uncomfortable, learning experience. Should a similar situation occur in the future I will be better equipped to deal with it more effectively as a part of a professional team rather than going off as a lone loose cannon.

CONCLUSION

The benefits of reflection have been explored in this chapter and also various methods of putting it into practice. Realistically, it may not always be possible to reflect on practice immediately after the event but this chapter has stressed the importance of finding a method which feels comfortable and then implementing it either individually or as a group. Allen (1985) sums up this importance as 'the advantage of critical social science for nursing and nurses is that it offers the opportunity to shatter the ideological mirror that traps us and our clients. It forces us to question that status quo at every turn' (p. 62). It is only by continually questioning that status quo that our nursing practice will be dynamic and not static.

REFERENCES

Allan, P. and Jolley, M. (eds) (1987) *The Curriculum in Nursing Education.* Croom Helm, London.

Allen, D. (1985) Nursing and social control: alternative models of science that emphasise understanding and emancipation. *Journal of Nursing Scholarship* 17(2): 58–64.

Alexander, M. (1982) Integrating theory and practice in nursing. *Nursing Times* 78(18): 68–71.

Allport, G.W. (1961) *Pattern and Growth in Personality.* Holt, Rinehart and Wilson, New York.

Argyle, J. (1983) *The Psychology of Interpersonal Behaviour*. Pelican, London.

Benner, P. (1984) *From Novice to Expert: excellence and power in clinical nursing practice*. Addison Wesley, California.

Brookfield, S. (1987) *Developing Critical Thinkers: challenging adults to explore alternative ways of thinking and acting*. Open University Press, Milton Keynes.

Burnard, P. (1985) *Learning Human Skills: a guide for nurses*. Heinemann, London.

Carper, B. (1978) Fundamental ways of knowing in nursing. *Advances in Nursing Science* 1(1): 13–23.

Cormack, D.F.S. (1983) *Psychiatric Nursing Described*. Churchill Livingstone, Edinburgh.

Crow, R. (1978) *The development of breast and bottle feeding in human infants*. PhD thesis, University of Edinburgh.

Cunningham, C.V. (1979) *Staff Nurses and Their Reasons for Leaving*. Master of Philosophy thesis, Edinburgh.

Darbyshire, P. (1993) In the hall of mirrors ... reflective practice. *Nursing Times* 89(49): 26–29.

Dewey, J. (1933) *Theory and Nature*. Dover, New York.

Dreyfus, J.L. and Dreyfus, S.E. (1985) *Mind Over Machine*. Free Press, New York.

Durgahee, T. (1996) Promoting reflection in post graduate nursing: a theoretical model. *Nurse Education Today* 16(6): 419–426.

Emden, C. (1991) Becoming a reflective practitioner. In: Grey, G. and Pratt, R. (Eds) *Towards a discipline of nursing*. Churchill Livingstone, Melbourne.

Erikson, E. (1963) *Childhood and Society*. W.W. Norton, New York.

Flanagan, J. (1954) The critical incident technique. *Psychological Bulletin* 51: 327–358.

Freud, S. (1961) *The Ego and the Id*. Hogarth Press, London.

Gormley, K.J. (1997) Practice write ups: an assessment instrument that contributes to bridging the differences between theory and practice for student nurses through the development of core skills. *Nurse Education Today* 17(1): 53–57.

Graham, I. (1995) Using structured reflection to improve nursing practice. *Nursing Times* 94(25): 56–59.

Greenwood, J. (1993) The reflective practice. *Journal of Advanced Nursing* 18: 1183–1187.

Jarvis, P. (1992) Reflective practice. *Nursing Education Today* 12: 174–181.

Johns, C. (1996) How the Burford reflective model boosts care standards. *Nursing Times* 92(36): 48–50.

Jung, C.G. (1978) *Man and His Symbols*. Picador, London.

Kohlberg, L. (1968) Moral development. In: *International Encyclopedia of Social Science*. Macmillan, New York.

Kolb, D. (1984) *Experimental Learning: experience as a source of learning and development*. Prentice Hall, New Jersey.

Laing, R.D. (1959) *The Divided Self*. Pelican, Harmondsworth.

Long, P. (1976) Judging and reporting on student nurse clinical performance: some problems for the ward sister. *International Journal of Nursing Studies*, 13: 115–121.

Lumby, J. (1991) *Nursing reflecting on an evolving practice*. Deakin University Press, Geelong, Victoria.

Mahler, M. (1975) *The Psychological Birth of the Human Infant*. Basic Books, New York.

Mead, G.H. (1934) *Mind, Self and Society*. University of Chicago Press, Chicago.

Minghella, E. and Benson, A. (1995) Developing reflective practice in mental health nursing through critical incident analysis. *Journal of Advanced Nursing* 21(2): 205–213.

Oliver, R.W. (1993) *Psychology and Health Care*. Baillière Tindall, London.

Palmer, A., Burns, S. and Bulman, C. (eds) (1994) *Reflective Practice in Nursing*. Blackwell Scientific Publications, Oxford.

Peplau, H.E. (1991) *Interpersonal Relations in Nursing*. Springer, New York.

Piaget, J. and Inhelder, B. (1969) *The Psychology of the Child*. Basic Books, New York.

Robinson, K. and Vaughan, B. (1992) *Knowledge for Nursing Practice*. Butterworth Heinemann, Oxford.

Rolfe, G. (1997) Beyond expertise: theory, practice and the reflective practitioner. *Journal of Clinical Nursing* 6(2): 93–97.

Sartre, J.P. (1956) *Being and Nothingness*. Philosophical Library, New York.

Schon, D. with Argyris, C. (1974) *Theory in Practice: increasing professional effectiveness*. Jossey Bass, New York.

Schon, D. (1987) *Educating the Reflective Practitioner*. Jossey Bass, New York.

Schon, D. (1991) *Educating the Reflective Practitioner*. Jossey Bass, Oxford.

Schon, D. (1995) *The Reflective Practitioner*. Jossey Bass, New York.

Sims, A. (1976) The critical incident technique in evaluating student nurse performance. *International Journal of Nursing Studies* 13(2): 123–130.

Street, A. (1991) *From Image to Action: Reflection in nursing practice*. Deakin University, Geelong, Victoria.

Sullivan, H.S. (1953) *The Independent Theory of Psychiatry*. W.W. Norton, New York.

Travelbee, J. (1971) *Interpersonal Aspects of Nursing*, 2nd edn. F.A. Davis, Philadelphia.

Van Manen, M. (1991) *The Tact of Teaching: the meaning of pedagogical thoughtfulness*. Free Press, New York.

6 THE NURSE AS MANAGER

Mohammed Abuel Ealeh and Rob Lancaster

OBJECTIVES

After reading this chapter, you should be able to:

- describe the key issues and concepts of management encompassed within the role of the mental health nurse
- demonstrate a good level of understanding and application of statutory requirements relating to the managerial role of the mental health nurse
- analyse the evolving managerial expectations of mental health nurses in the light of the changing contexts in which they work
- critique the role of the mental health nurse as a manager of the multidisciplinary team within inpatient and community-based settings
- reflect on your own performance as a manager through reflective practice and clinical supervision.

INTRODUCTION

Mental health nurses remain the largest part of the workforce in mental health care. As has been shown in the previous chapters, both the context and content of their work have changed dramatically. The management structures, style and functions have had to adapt with the shift to community mental health care. At the same time there have been radical shifts in the way people think about management as a practice, in questioning both its role and value within organizations.

Historically mental health nursing managers were concerned with ensuring the smooth running of the mental hospitals. The responsibility for the overall institution would be shared between the most senior nurse (e.g. chief male nurse), a senior psychiatrist (physician superintendent) and an administrator (hospital secretary). The environment would be fairly predictable and the demands of the workforce largely unchanging.

Under these conditions the tasks of managers would be concerned with maintaining the system. Most activity within the institution would be prescribed by procedure and policy. Widespread standardization would be found within hospitals and similarities would exist between hospitals. An emphasis was placed upon containment and order. Divisions of labour were tightly circumscribed. Whilst the institutional care which was the norm until relatively recently has been criticized, it should be realized that the ideology behind the development of the mental hospital system was essentially benign. Although now unacceptable in clinical and ethical terms, the operation of the institution was based upon a theoretical view of the needs of the patients. Patients would directly benefit from the stability, routine and order of the hospital. Criticism of this system and particular hospitals led to efforts to optimize the conditions rather than examine the underlying principles. Until recently, no significant discourse existed to describe alternatives. The management task was to sustain this system. The management can be seen as both a contributor to and product of the regime. Clearly defined hierarchies existed within the nursing profession with a clear differentiation between ward-based staff and 'management'. The culture of the mental hospital was such that the system was seen to be more important than the staff within it who were by and large interchangeable.

In terms of context, management within mental health nursing has to take into account the major shift which has taken place from hospital to community settings and the major reforms which the NHS itself has undergone.

The central element of the reforms led to the introduction of the purchaser/provider split and the creation of competition between NHS trusts for available business. For mental health service provision, and therefore mental health nursing, there is an added element. As a direct result of the reforms, a substantial part of current mental health provision is now provided within the independent sector including both the private and voluntary sectors and this too has significant implications for nurses holding supervisory and managerial roles. The NHS reforms and the resultant changes occurred during the last 20 years and were driven by the previous Conservative governments. The effects of these reforms and changes, however, continued after the Conservatives lost office to Labour in May 1997. Moreover, the Labour government, which itself is thirsty for reform, is planning to introduce yet more change in mental health policy and provision. The overall effect is that things have become extremely complex and the relative stability which characterized the 1960s and 1970s has given way to instability, confusion and much uncertainty.

Contemporary management concepts in mental health nursing centre around widely accepted ideas such as multidisciplinary teams and multiagency working, good enough clinical knowledge of mental health problems, treatment approaches, team leadership, management of change, collaboration and partnership, including that with mental health service users, and clinical supervision. Also any consideration of the role of the mental health nurse as a manager must include establishing a confident knowledge base of essential information relating to statutory requirements and relevant legal issues and their implications.

Nurses continue to constitute the largest proportion of workers of any mental health team whether this is based in inpatient or community settings and regardless of whether this is within the NHS or the private sector. It is also true that nurses continue to be the only type of health worker in frequent, intimate and prolonged contact with clients and their carers. Moreover, whilst medical staff continue to have medical responsibility for clients, they still have to rely to a large extent on nurses for the assessment of clients' mental health problems, the implementation of treatment programmes prescribed and the monitoring of the effectiveness of such treatment. Furthermore, mental health nurses working in inpatient settings continue to play the key role in coordinating the contribution of different health and social care workers involved in the care programme of clients under their care, as well as forming the link connecting such clients with other clients, relatives and carers. As Wright (1993) argued, nurses have the greatest influence on how resources are spent on patients, and can affect the quality of patient care more significantly than any other single professional group.

Much of the nurse's work is about management, whether she is engaged in catering for the diverse needs of a range of different clients in community settings, managing a ward full of patients, is in charge of a particular locality, unit or holding a more senior post. It is therefore very important for mental health nurses to understand key management concepts and what they entail and to develop their managerial skills.

However, prequalifying nursing education, including mental health nursing, has not historically equipped them to be managers and generally speaking, they were promoted to supervisory roles because of their clinical or practice skills (Forrest 1983). The need for better preparation for managerial roles has been emphasized by many nurse authors and government reports (Forrest 1983, King's Fund 1981, Ministry of Health SHHD 1966, Rowden 1987). There is also an acknowledged shortage of professional leaders within mental health nursing. This was highlighted in the 1994 review of mental health nursing (DoH 1994) which emphasized the need to incorporate skills in general management and leadership into nurse training so that nursing qualifications could be seen as a firm basis for management development.

This chapter is intentionally written from the perspective of both the manager and the team she manages. The reader is seen as a manager and a member of a team within the grand scheme of things. Moreover, managers do not practise in a vacuum; at least they are not supposed to do so! Whilst attempting to cover all essential aspects of management and their application to mental health nursing, this chapter is written from a practical and realistic perspective. Much of the focus is on everyday issues and the challenges that face nurse managers in different context. Whilst alluding to the work of key management authors as well as mental health nursing leaders and academics and utilizing the language of management as and when appropriate, the intention is to ensure that the contents are relevant, practicable, accessible and hopefully interesting.

In structuring this chapter, we have striven to strike a balance between management theory and policy. In keeping with the overall style of this book, we have included two case studies; the first is intended to illustrate the role of the CPA key worker and the other demonstrates management of change in action and the real world.

KEY ISSUES AND CONCEPTS OF MANAGEMENT

There are many ways of defining management. The simplest and perhaps the most succinct is to view management as getting the work done through others. However, the connoisseur may well be aggrieved at this broad-brush approach. She may wish to highlight a whole range of concepts including: establishing aims and objectives, standards and targets; planning and organizing the means of achieving these; monitoring and controlling the process of achieving these aims; and reviewing results, developing staff, structures and systems. She may further wish to emphasize the need for motivating staff, good decision making skills, effective communication, sensitivity and persuasion skills.

But then, this chapter is not especially for connoisseurs. Rather, it is a focused effort, practicable and is intentionally user friendly. Readers who wish to delve deeper into the whole range of management concepts are referred to the list of references and suggested further reading at the end of the chapter. We have selected a number of key issues which we regard as the most relevant and these will now be discussed in some detail.

Management and leadership

It is rare to discuss management without including the concept of leadership. The debate is complex and there is much overlap and interdependence between the two. Mintzberg (1973) suggested that leadership is but one aspect of the managerial job. Management may be seen to be primarily concerned with everyday matters, routine but important work and organization of resources of which people are a part. Leadership, on the other hand, may be considered to be more concerned with change and innovation and leading the teams and individual members who will deliver a given task or carry out a certain function. It is also suggested that enhanced leadership effectiveness does increase organizational effectiveness (House 1988).

However, even though management is not leadership, many managers are also leaders and good leaders are likely to manage things more effectively and to achieve better results. Effective management requires knowledge, competence, cooperation by the workers and satisfaction from customers (clients). The many elements which constitute management and the numerous qualities and facets desired by leaders indicate that a well-rounded person is required. However, Handy (1985) reminds us that one can be so well rounded as to have no edges left to cut with! As in many matters, balance is all important. Despite the many leadership theories and models on offer, we have yet to develop approaches to leadership which actually help managers to increase their effectiveness (Tetrault *et al.* 1988). Similarly, whilst the leadership arena is replete with conceptualizations and empirical investigations, few authors have been concerned with developing 'hands-on' approaches to leadership effectiveness.

Management/leadership style

Style is another key issue that management commentators refer to and they are not generally talking about the type of clothes that people are wearing! However, dress codes could be highly relevant when considering the culture of an organization. Style refers to how people carry out their management and leadership roles and some styles may be more effective under differing circumstances.

An enduring and fundamental distinction has been drawn between democratic and autocratic approaches. Essentially, *autocratic* approaches are likely to be underpinned by an authoritarian view that 'people are dependent, indolent, self-centred and uncooperative. People are assumed to need strong direction and control by external forces if discipline is to be maintained' (Maier and Hayes 1962 in Vroom and Deci 1974). This view parallels MacGregor's 'Theory X' which assumes that the average person dislikes work and will seek to avoid it where possible, most people need to be controlled and threatened before they will perform effectively and most people prefer to be led, dislike responsibility, are lacking in ambition and like and need security above all else (MacGregor 1960). By contrast, *democratic* approaches are underpinned by a view that '(men) work harder when left to themselves and are allowed to have a say in what happens' (Argyle *et al.* 1958 in Vroom and Deci 1974). This view parallels MacGregor's 'Theory Y' which assumes that the effort people put into their work is natural, man is capable of self-direction if he is committed to the objectives of the organization and the job is satisfying, punishment and control are not necessarily the only way to make people perform well, people can learn and accept as well as seek responsibility on a personal level, creativity and imagination are essential aspects and may be used to solve problems at work, and we rarely fully utilize the capabilities of the average worker. A combination of MacGregor's theories X and Y was proposed by Ouchi (1981) who sensibly suggested that people can have characteristics attributed to both theories X and Y rather than just one or the other. In Ouchi's theory Z, involvement of all employees is valued and the manager is seen as responsible for creating an environment in which there is a philosophy of mutual commitment, and continued development of the individual (Rocchiccioli and Tilbury 1998).

There is a relationship between style and context. More recent theorists have emphasized the need for flexibility in style according to the situation and the characteristics of the staff group. The manager who can employ a range of styles is the most effective. This is not to be confused with inconsistency or unpredictability where no one can tell how a manager is going to behave from one day to the next. Fiedler developed the theory of contingency management where style needs to vary according to the situation. For example, task-focused approaches can work well where there is a poor structure. Hersey and Blanchard (1982) related style to the maturity of the staff group in terms of their knowledge, skills and motivation. Immature groups require a highly task-focused style which can change to a more socially focused style as the group matures.

Zarod defined four styles which need to be harnessed in order to produce effective management. These are directive, supportive, coaching and delegating. *Directive* approaches may be effective but can limit staff involvement and cause motivation to fade. The *supportive* approach will involve 'giving staff the time and space to take on new roles, offering them support, listening to them, and motivating them for a given period'. *Coaching* moves people to take up new roles or skills. This can be time consuming but in the long term can bring many benefits. Finally, *delegation* is a highly evolved style of management that must be accompanied by careful planning and the ability to maintain a skilful overview. The effective manager needs to know when to use what approach and with which people.

Organizational structure

Structure is concerned with how an organization defines responsibilities through a chain of command and with the relationships of different components and functions of one another. It is often depicted through an organizational chart *organogram*. On its own a good structure will not guarantee success but poor structure will almost always guarantee failure.

Structure should not be considered without also looking at the concept of organizational culture. We have become used to regular changes in structures within NHS trusts and within the wider organization of the NHS (e.g. the purchaser/provider spilt). Reorganization or, as the cynics call it, re-disorganization has become a way of life. The primary aim of such structural change is to improve the effectiveness of the organization.

Over time different types of structure become more popular and organizations may be moving between different models, e.g. from divisional to functional or from centralized to decentralized. In recent times, the most significant direction has been towards flatter structures with less hierarchy. The themes of empowerment and downsizing have accompanied this. Clarke (1994) has described four types of organization.

- *The flat organization* – this involves sweeping away layers of management and departments and allocating resources to support the 'front line' which deals with the customer. Underpinning this process is a view that layers of management impede communications and become self-serving rather than being customer oriented.
- *The customer-centred organization* – this type of organization develops its structure to reflect different markets rather than functions.
- *The network organization* – this emphasizes developing the effectiveness of horizontal rather than vertical processes. Everyone is someone else's customer and there is an emphasis on promoting effectiveness across functional boundaries.
- *The cellular organization* – this 'consists of a collection of small teams, each with a high degree of autonomy'. Each cell may be responsible for most aspects of business with no central departments. 'Each member of the

team has a high sense of ownership and responsibility for the team's output' (Clarke 1994).

As with style, different types of structures may suit different activities so that even within one organization variation may be found. Leavitt (1964 in Vroom and Deci 1974) suggested that for programmed repetitive tasks, highly centralized communication structures seem to operate most efficiently but with some human costs. Where the task is less structured, more open communication nets with larger numbers of channels and less differentiation among members seem to work more effectively.

Organizational culture

When describing or attempting to analyse organizations there are two recurrent concepts to consider: structure and culture. Whilst structure determines how the organization or service arranges its plants, personnel and divisions, culture is an altogether more 'slippery' notion. These days structures may last no more than 2–3 years before they are reorganized in a continual effort to improve performance and keep up with competitors. Nevertheless, structural solutions may be overvalued as a response to what may be primarily cultural obstacles to change.

Handy (1985) provides a highly accessible description of culture and a model of categorization. He defines culture as sets of values and beliefs, conveying more of a feeling of pervasive way of life or set of norms. These beliefs extend to the way in which work should be organized, authority exercised, people rewarded and/or controlled. Further features concern the levels of formalization, degree of planning required and the ways in which initiatives from subordinates are viewed. Handy argued that within the same organizations different cultures may be found.

Handy described four types of organizational culture: power, role, task and person. The *power* culture depends on a centralized figure with power emanating from the centre in a web-like fashion. There may be fewer rules or procedures and little bureaucracy. By contrast, the *role* culture is often stereotyped as bureaucracy with a role or job being more important than the individual who fills it. The efficiency of this culture depends upon the rationality of allocation of work and responsibility rather than on the individual's competencies. The *task* culture is job or project orientated with an emphasis on getting things done. 'The outcome of the team's work tends to be the common enemy, obliterating individual objectives and most status and style differences' (p. 182). The *person* culture revolves around the individual and any structure is seen to exist in order to assist him or her. Such cultures are rare and may only be found in highly professionalized areas or where the employee's skills are highly sought after by others. Individuals may feel only loosely affiliated to the organization and may be difficult to influence.

Different cultures may be able to cope better with different activities, including responding to change. Schein (1984) proposed a more dynamic model of organizational culture with different layers. Most evident are those artefacts such as dress, technology and office layout. Next are those values which underpin behaviour which include espoused or manifest values. This level must be penetrated to grasp the 'underlying assumptions' which are generally unconscious but which ultimately determine how people think, feel and behave.

Understanding the significance of culture and its often unconscious manifestation is crucial for not only managers but any staff member who is grappling with introducing an improvement in the service, no matter how small. Both Schein and Handy view the adaptation of culture as being crucial to the organization's survival. Change may be painful and elicit strong resistance and, as Schein (1984) argued, 'may not even be possible without replacing the large numbers of people who wish to hold on to all of the original culture'.

Coordination and management of care

Coordination and management of all aspects of care to different clients is an important role of the nurse manager. Whether the nurse is acting as a ward manager, primary nurse or a CPA key worker, the coordinator role is essential. Coordination relates to assessment and the delivery and monitoring of clients' care plans, different aspects of care provided by different mental health workers including nurses, medical staff, psychologists, occupational therapists and others, client's views of their care plan, the views of their carers and relatives and of the formal care team.

Despite the importance of this role, it is often overlooked or is taken for granted by both nurse colleagues and other team members. Effective coordination is smooth and seamless so it can go unnoticed and may therefore be undervalued. Yet coordination is one of the most sophisticated aspects of the role of the nurse manager. It requires liaison, negotiation and political skills. The mental health nurse manager's role is to engender the support and enthusiasm of people who are in different positions of power and authority, including those below and above her in the hierarchy. This further requires gaining the respect and confidence of different team members and attaining a respectable degree of knowledge and expertise not only of her own domain but also a broad perspective of those of other team members.

Expertise

Clients and their relatives, junior colleagues and nursing students, other professional colleagues and relevant authorities reasonably expect the mental health nurse acting as manager to have attained a considerable degree of expertise in mental health care and work with clients in different settings, essential aspects of legislation, administrative skills, liaison and management of both human and other resources. The translation of this expertise into everyday practice means that the nurse manager is expected to demonstrate competence in a diverse range of situations. These include welcoming, settling and reassuring disturbed clients and worried relatives, ability to undertake various therapeutic intervention skills, creating and maintaining a positive ward climate conducive to individualized care for clients and effective learning for students, effective management of staff and other resources.

The issue of what kind of knowledge should underpin the education and training of mental health nurses has exercised the minds of many and it remains the subject of debate. The current emphasis on people with serious and enduring mental illness, for example, is thought to be politically driven by government whose policies and guidelines since the mid-1990s are viewed as an expedient and belated response to the failure of community care (Barker 1998). Nevertheless, mental health nurses working in different contexts and settings are required to adapt their practice to this emphasis. This is not unusual since, as has been shown in other chapters in this book, mental health nurses have always had to adapt their roles and their practice to the changing demands of external forces. The authors believe, however, that investment of self in order to help others in distress will remain the key human activity which characterizes the mental health nurse's role. This is what mental health service users continue to say they want from psychiatric services; ordinary human responses, interaction and support (Rogers *et al.* 1993). To this end, the role of the manager is to harness the knowledge, expertise and energies of team members and mobilize them in order to help clients and their relatives.

Communication

The ward manager is expected to liaise with many people on a daily basis. She needs to know her team and to gain their confidence and respect. She needs to be friendly and approachable, able to inspire her colleagues and to be at ease in her many capacities. she needs to be able to 'role her sleeves up and muck in when necessary' but without shying away from taking tough decisions and resolving difficult problems when she has to.

Team members appreciate 'hard-working' managers and ones who lead from the front and by example. More recent management rhetoric values managers who work 'smarter' rather than harder. The reality in many ward or team settings is that team members are stressed out of their minds trying to ensure that all necessary tasks are completed on time. The successful manager is one who can ease out some of this stress and motivate her colleagues to achieve their targets and manage their workload reasonably well. Successful team leaders can create a positive atmosphere, even in difficult circumstances, in which team members feel valued and supported and in which communication channels flow freely and smoothly.

Effective leadership also facilitates and encourages reflection. This involves ongoing examination and analysis of the objectives of the team, the extent to which these are being achieved, open communication about successful strategies and those which did not work out and learning from the experience as a whole. Working in complex settings such as those in the mental health arena is very demanding. It can also form a barrier to effective communication. There are, of course, many other barriers to communication ranging from the obvious, such as language difficulties and poor record keeping, for example, to the less visible such as negative attitudes and stereotyping by the team members themselves. These need to be recognized by the mental health nurse manager so that she can combat the possibility by the provision of appropriate support mechanisms to facilitate and enhance team effectiveness.

Resource management

Effective management is concerned, among many other things, with the optimum utilization of resources (Johns and Graham 1994). Whether functioning at a ward, locality or directorate level, the nurse manager's role includes important management of human and other resources. In the context of mental health nursing, one of the main challenges is concerned with ensuring adequate, fair and appropriate allocation of staff. This is increasingly becoming a major problem. Serious shortages of mental health nurses – made worse by poor manpower planning in the early and mid-1990s when the numbers of students contracted for were cut and by recurring recruitment difficulties at present – compound this problem. Team members are the most important resource and effective team working is the key to achieving organizational objectives.

Time is a precious commodity and a scarce resource. Nurses frequently complain about lack of time or not having enough time to do this or that task. Whether in inpatient or community settings, mental health nurses often complain about the amount of time they have to spend on paperwork. Procrastination, perfectionism and lack of prioritization are the enemies of effective time management (Marelli 1993). Successful mental health nurse managers anticipate, plan and prioritize their workload. They can organize their paperwork, make wise use of technology such as email, are assertive and sensitive to their own needs as well as those of their team members. There are many books and manuals which can help the mental health nurse manager to learn how to be more effective through time management (for example, Blanchard and Johnson 1983, Forsyth 1994, Masterton 1997).

Delegation

Effective managers delegate. Management, as indicated earlier, is about getting the work done through others. Delegation, however, is not easy. Many managers appear convinced that if a job is worth doing well then they must do it themselves and that it will not be done as well if someone else does it! This is not just about arrogance or an inflated sense of self-importance, but a genuine fear or worry that the surest way of doing things well is to do them yourself. However, the effective manager is able to make the best use of her team members, knowing their strengths and weaknesses, knowing the 'cart horse' from the 'race horse' and delegating various tasks accordingly.

Effective management is about maintaining a broader perspective on things whilst remaining in touch with the finest details. It is about utilizing what has come to be known as the helicopter effect, hovering over the situation and maintaining an overview, but remaining in close touch with members of the team. The Audit Commission recognized the multiple responsibilities of the role of the nurse manager and the pressures associated with this role. This emphasizes the importance of delegation (Koontz and Weihrich 1988), letting go of the responsibilities and entrusting team members with them.

Decision making

Decision making in today's ever-changing mental health-care settings is more complex. The need is for creativity, flexibility and ability to respond rapidly. Tensions and conflicts within community mental health teams often complicate the picture further. Changing government priorities and policies, the demands for evidence-based practice, service user involvement, greater transparency and clinical governance are among the many external factors and pressures that exert major influence on the process of decision making. Vroom and Vetton (1973) developed a decision tree (Box 6.1) which may be helpful in understanding the process of decision making at different levels. It is worth noting that the lower down the tree a decision is made, the more empowering the leadership style and the environment in which it operates.

Managing change

Managers in all types of organizations, including mental health care contexts, and at all levels are confronted with an unprecedented amount of change and turmoil. Understanding the processes of change, instigating change, acting as a change agent, implementing change and monitoring the effectiveness of change implemented have all come to be a part of the mental health nurse manager's job. Change has also become an instrument or a kind of a yardstick by which the effectiveness of managers is measured.

Change and its many aspects and variables have become extremely difficult to predict. The American management guru Tom Peters and his many followers have become preoccupied with change and its implications for organizations. So much so, that he went as far as suggesting that the only criterion for success is

---

Box 6.1   Vroom and Vetton (1973) decision tree

Decisions may be reached in one of the following ways.

- The leader makes a decision without consulting anyone and assumes full accountability.
- The leader makes a decision after informally consulting one or two people in the organization.
- The leader makes a decision after convening a task force to analyse the problem.
- The leader makes a decision following a committee report.
- The leader asks a committee to consult, produce and publish a report, to decide on a solution and agrees to support their decision.

'Are you changing enough, rapidly enough, to successfully confront the future?' (Peters 1988). Whilst Tom Peters may be primarily concerned with commercial organizations, his underlying thinking and principles do apply to other contexts, including those in which mental health nurses work. Nurse managers who have witnessed or even played a part in the many and frequent changes in their working environment during the last two decades will identify with Peters' assertion that 'If you are not reorganizing, pretty substantially, once every six to twelve months, you are probably out of step with the times'! Change by itself, on the other hand, is neither good nor bad, it is inevitable (White 1998). Mental health nurse managers have to face the challenge change presents and it is planned change that is the main concern here. There are many other concepts associated with change and we will be discussing some of these later in this chapter. The classic change theory of Kurt Lewin (1951) is widely known and continues to be used in explaining the change process. This, together with the Bennis *et al.* (1985) change strategies, will be discussed later.

Developing management competence

It is important to involve as many people as possible in the overall management process for a clinical team or department. There are two key reasons for this. First, it is essential to promote maximum ownership of policy initiatives and any clinical innovations. Second, it is vital to ensure an even distribution of some management competence in all members of a team.

The first point could be summarized by the apparently contradictory maxim that 'management is too important to be left to the managers!' There is a real danger in developing policy or change programmes in isolation, releasing them upon a team and then becoming frustrated at the extent of difficulty in implementing new policies or changes. There are hazards of creating a climate of change fatigue. People working in human services can become demoralized at the pace and frequency of change. This can lead to widespread disaffection. Top-down approaches, characterized by central diktat and bureaucracy, will result in alienation and resistance. These can be reduced, if not always eliminated, by routinely involving front-line practitioners in service development. Such staff have the most contact with service users and are best placed to contribute to policy and procedural changes. They will understand the implications for the team as a whole and for the service user. Managers may feel that change is their own domain but they cling to this view at their peril. Delegation of decision making needs to be balanced against the possibility that some practitioners may take a parochial view and may prefer to carry on doing things in the same way.

Second, developing a wider degree of management competence in a team just makes good sense. The location of power, decision making and influence in one or a few individuals can be dangerous. In such a climate if a manager leaves or is off sick then a team can become rudderless and feel resentful. It is unhealthy for people to work in a climate where there is repeated deference to a manager or managers. By delegating and dispersing managerial authority, practitioners can make a wider contribution to the service. This can be achieved in a number of ways. For example, the involvement of junior staff or students in time-limited projects can bring much needed clinical perspectives to the management process and improve levels of confidence in those participating. Junior staff must be allowed to make mistakes on occasions and invariably there will be greater commitment where staff believe that they have driven the change rather merely being victims of it. This should be done in a meaningful and genuine way rather than through manipulation or abdication of responsibility.

Another way in which management competence can be developed is through deputizing and shadowing arrangements. Appraisals and performance reviews provide a forum for identifying how this can be achieved.

MENTAL HEALTH POLICY

Current legislation: the Mental Health Act 1983

It is not our intention here to provide the customary section on the Mental Health Act 1983 since there are many sources which serve this purpose. These include the Act itself and the *Code of Practice: Mental Health Act 1983* (DoH and Welsh Office 1993). It is recognized, however, that an accurate understanding of the Act constitutes an important part of the role of the mental health nurse manager. It is also essential to know how to find out the finer details. At the time of writing, the Act itself is subject to review and major changes are anticipated. Accordingly, rather than presenting the different parts and sections of the Act, we provide a brief critique and update of relevant issues emanating from or relating to the Act and planned legislation.

Whilst the Act was seen by many to have enhanced the rights of mental health service users and extended care in the community for a large number of patients, others saw it as contributing to a series of problems experienced by many users and to have had a major negative impact on the community at large. The new (Labour) Secretary of State for Health, Frank Dobson, declared in July 1998 that 'Care in the community has failed'. In a written answer to a parliamentary question, Mr Dobson stated that:

> *The law on mental health is based on the needs and therapies of a bygone age. Its revision in 1983 merely tinkered with the problem. What I want now is a root and branch review to reflect the opportunities and limits of modern therapies and drugs. It will cover such possible measures as compliance orders and community treatment orders to provide a prompt and effective legal basis to ensure that patients get supervised care if they do not take their medication or if their condition deteriorates.*

More recent statements and utterances by Mr Dobson have further indicated that there is likely to be clearer guidance and directives with regard to people with personality disorders. The document *Modernising Mental Health Services: safe, sound and supportive* (DoH 1998) points out that:

The Mental Health Act has also failed to provide an adequate framework for dealing with a quite different group of people; those with severe antisocial personality disorder who present a risk to the public. Shortcomings in the Mental Health Act, coupled with failures to provide proper continuity of care after discharge from hospital, have led to terrible consequences in some tragic cases.

Accordingly, the stage is set for major changes to come, and whilst these will not be implemented overnight, mental health nurse managers have to recognize the new climate and its likely implications. And although there are many supporters of the changes, some of whom have actively and successfully campaigned for them in recent times, there are many opposing views too. Rather than indulging in the debate, we believe it is more useful to contemplate the National Service Framework introduced by the Government in the Spring of 1999, and to explore the action plan for developing safe, sound and supportive mental health services. Figure 6.1 below illustrates the details.

New and added emphasis is to be placed on more prompt assessment, risk management, early intervention, home treatment and assertive outreach. These will be complemented by forensic and secure provision. Progress achieved in recent times in terms of service user and carer involvement as well as collaboration and partnership among the different agencies involved in mental health-care provision will continue. In contemplating the new rhetoric, mental health nurse managers will no doubt wonder whether this is merely old wine in new bottles. A more positive view of the planned changes, however, may be to see them as providing a more up-to-date and comprehensive service for people with mental health problems and a long overdue process of facing the challenges and real dangers that a minority of individuals with severe mental disorder have caused to both themselves and the community at large.

The 1983 Act is seen to be more concerned with hospital-based treatment and is no longer applicable in an era when much of mental health care provision is based in the community. The team of experts reviewing the Mental Health Act

SAFE	SOUND	SUPPORTIVE
Good risk management	24 hour access	Involvement of patients, service users and carers
Early intervention	Needs assessment	Access to employment, education and housing
Enough beds	Good primary care	Working in partnership
Better outreach	Effective treatment	Better information
Integrated forensic and secure provision	Effective care processes	Promoting good mental health and reducing stigma

A modern legislative framework

Figure 6.1   Action Plan for Safe, Sound and Supportive Mental Health Services, DoH (1998)

1983 reported in the summer of 1999, and this review provides the basis for legislation for the new millennium. The new Government is clearly concerned about and committed to enacting new legislation specifically directed at those who are considered to have severe anti-social personality disorder. The Government is proposing to create 'a new form of reviewable detention for those people with a severe personality disorder who are considered to pose a grave risk to the public' (DoH 1998).

We now turn our attention, albeit briefly, to other important aspects of mental health legislation and guidelines which pertain to the daily work of mental health nurses and managers.

The Care Programme Approach

The origins of the Care Programme Approach (CPA) may be traced to the Spokes Report (DoH 1989). However, an earlier report by the Social Services Select Committee (1985) had recommended that:

> *Nobody should be discharged from hospital without a practical individual care plan jointly devised by all concerned, communicated to all those responsible for its implementation and with a mechanism for monitoring its implementation ... and that the resources for this be made available.*

The Spokes Report made three recommendations which may be seen to have led to the introduction of the CPA in 1991. These were:

- that health authorities (HAs) and local authorities (LAs) and relevant voluntary organizations should jointly provide aftercare for informal ex-psychiatric patients until they reached a joint decision that it was no longer required
- that, prior to discharge, individual community care plans should be prepared which include a day for review
- that multidisciplinary care for patients should be promoted.

Although the 1989 White Paper *Caring for People* required all HAs, in collaboration with Social Services authorities, to introduce the CPA from April 1991 and despite further guidance issued in September 1990, many authorities did not introduce the CPA until much later. Clinicians were not particularly keen to comply with the requirements of the CPA which were considered to be cumbersome and bureaucratic. The DoH responded by introducing the notion of tiered CPA, with three levels of user need generating three levels of responses from minimal to full CPA.

The essential elements of the CPA as outlined in HSG(94)27 are:

- a care plan agreed between the relevant professional staff, the patient, his or her carers and recorded in writing
- the allocation of a key worker and regular review of the patient's progress and health and social care needs.

The DoH continued to emphasize the importance of the CPA and its adoption. So much so that the 1996 document *Building Bridges* (DoH 1996b) stated that 'The CPA is the cornerstone of the government's mental health policy. It applies to all mentally ill patients who are accepted by the specialist mental health services'.

Care management

About the same time that the DoH imposed the CPA upon health authorities, it also required local authorities to introduce care management (DoH 1991a, b). The essential stages of care management are (Kane *et al.* 1991):

- screening
- assessment
- care planning
- implementation
- monitoring
- reassessment

HSG(94)27 makes it clear that Social Services Departments (SSDs) have duties under the NHS and Community Care Act 1990 to assess people's needs for community care services. Some of the guidance was rather conflicting in that it stated that 'Multidisciplinary assessment under the CPA will fulfil these duties' and 'One way of looking at the CPA is as a specialist variant of care management for people with mental health problems, and the two systems should be capable of being fully integrated with one another (DoH 1996b).

Supervision registers

Supervision registers were introduced against a background of media coverage of lapses in community care for people with serious mental illness, e.g. Christopher Clunis (Ritchie *et al.* 1994). The plan for introducing supervision registers was criticized by some psychiatrists as poorly thought out (Hunt 1994) and as policy making on the hoof. The guidelines for implementation were issued in February 1994 with a target date for implementation of 1st October 1994. Clients considered appropriate for inclusion on supervision registers are those suffering from severe mental illness who are liable to be at a significant risk of committing serious violence or suicide or of severe self-neglect.

A study by Davis and Woolgroove in 1998 involving 27 local English authorities, 137 social workers and 235 clients found that by the end of April 1996, a total of 2829 people were on the supervision register nationwide. This figure is considered to be less than the actual numbers because 36 out of the 190 NHS trust did not provide their figures. Of note is that 71% were male and 29% female. However, women made up only 19% of those listed as being at risk of violence, 35% of severe self-neglect and 43% at risk of suicide.

THE MENTAL HEALTH (PATIENTS IN THE COMMUNITY) ACT 1995

The Mental Health (Patients in the Community) Act 1995 received Royal Assent in November 1995, and came into effect on 1st April 1996. It complements

Table 6.1 Risk categorization of the 235 service users

Category of risk	No. of cases	%
Violence to others	82	35
Severe self-neglect	54	23
Suicide	23	10
Violence and self-neglect	41	17
Suicide and violence	17	7
Suicide and self-neglect	9	4
All three categories	9	4
All violence	149	63
All severe self-neglect	113	48
All suicide	56	24

supervision registers and reflects the Care Programme Approach. The 1995 Act is intended for the limited number of patients who, after being detained in hospital for treatment under the 1983 Mental Health Act, need formal supervision to ensure they receive suitable aftercare. The purpose of the Act is to help ensure that the client receives the aftercare services to be provided under Section (117) of the 1983 Act.

Before a client is discharged from hospital, a risk assessment must be carried out. A care plan is then established based on a systematic assessment of need and a key worker identified to monitor the client's progress and the delivery of care in the community. The services thus provided should then be kept under regular review in the light of the client's needs.

The new powers apply to those clients presenting a substantial risk of serious harm to the health and safety of themselves or of other people or of being seriously exploited if they do not receive suitable aftercare and as such they should normally be included on supervision registers. RMOs making an application for supervision orders must have satisfied themselves that the above conditions have been met *and* that supervision is likely to ensure that the client receives the necessary aftercare services.

The 1995 Act introduced three new provisions.

Table 6.2 Clinical diagnosis of patients on the supervision register

Diagnosis	Number	%
Schizophrenic illness	160	68
Paranoid/delusional	4	2
Affective disorders	39	17
Drug/alcohol induced	7	3
Dementia	4	2
Psychopathy/personality disorder	13	5
Other mental illness	8	3

1. A new power of supervised discharge for previously detained patients discharged into the community, to ensure that they stay in contact with services and cooperate with the aftercare plan that has been arranged for them.
2. The possibility of allowing detained patients to be given leave of absence from hospital under medical supervision for a longer period, to help them achieve a smoother transition to living outside a hospital environment.
3. Strengthening of the provisions for returning patients who go absent from hospital without leave.

The 1995 Act defines requirements which may be imposed when a patient is subject to supervised discharge. These are that the client should live in a particular place and attend a particular place at set times for medical treatment, occupation, education or training. However, the requirement to attend for medical treatment *does not* carry with it any power to impose medication or other treatment against the client's wishes! The supervisor, or person authorized by the supervisor, should be allowed access to the patient at his or her place of residence. The supervisor is responsible for monitoring the supervised discharge arrangements and for liaising with other members of the community team and coordinating their work where necessary. The supervisor also has the power to take and convey clients to a place where they are required to reside or to attend for medical treatment, occupation or training. The Act did not contain new powers to use 'unreasonable force' and no power to coerce the client into accepting medication or treatment.

ROLE OF THE CPA KEY WORKER

The aims of the Care Programme Approach and the role of the CPA key worker have been defined above. The role of the CPA key worker is critical in ensuring that the necessary care and treatment inputs are effectively provided for people with mental health problems to improve quality of life and to prevent people slipping through the net of care.

This section considers the tasks of the CPA key worker from a management perspective. The reader will be introduced to some of the managerial components of this role. This section assumes an adequate level of competence of care which needs to be aligned in order to produce and deliver an individualized care programme. A false dichotomy may exist between practice and service management which may impede an integrated approach to service development. Practice staff may see management as someone else's business. Front-line practice staff need to adopt a wide perspective of their work in order to understand and exploit the relationship between providing individual care and service development. The experiences and knowledge of the clientele that practice staff possess must be harnessed in order to drive improvements and changes in services. The management competencies defined here are:

- understanding of relevant policy and legislative changes
- communication, coordination and leadership within the multidisciplinary team
- utilizing resources and contributing to service planning
- organization of self and others; priority setting
- recognizing training needs
- use of clinical supervision.

CASE STUDY 6.1

John Boucher is a 44-year-old man who has been diagnosed as having a schizophrenic illness. Until recently he lived in a local authority flat with his mother who was of considerable support to him. Mrs Boucher had a stroke and was no longer able to look after the home or herself. She moved into residential care and John was left on his own in the flat. He had been difficult to engage in services since his initial breakdown but his more extreme symptoms had been controlled with depot medication which he grudgingly accepted from his CPN. His mother had prepared meals, cleaned the house, shopped and generally supported John with all activities of daily living. Following his mother's departure, John became increasingly reluctant to accept his medications and refused to accept any domiciliary support or attend any day services. He became markedly suspicious of his neighbours who complained to the housing department and he became abusive to the staff in the home where his mother now resided, believing that they had kidnapped her.

Eventually he was admitted to hospital under Section (3) of the 1983 Mental Health Act. He began to accept medication, his more positive symptoms began to subside and discharge was considered. He expressed a strong wish to return to his home and recognized that he would need to accept greater levels of support upon discharge. John accepted the appointment of his CPN as his CPA key worker. Short periods of leave were commenced during which John accepted visits from a support worker and attended the local day service for occupational therapy.

Understanding of relevant policy and legislative areas

Following admission under Section (3) both the health authority and social services are obliged to provide aftercare under Section (117). Consideration should be given to the use of Section (25 – Supervised Discharge) and placement on the supervision register. Assessment of risk needs to be undertaken given the potential for threatening behaviour towards others. Under the tiered approach to CPA, John comes into level two category and will require a formal multidisciplinary approach to care planning.

Communication, coordination and leadership within the multidisciplinary team

The CPA key worker should ensure that a care planning meeting takes place. Representatives of the health trust, including the RMO, and social services department should attend owing to the statutory requirements under Section (117). Local arrangements may vary for observing the requirements of the CPA and Section (117) but the basic principles remain the same and consideration should be given to streamlining the process and minimizing the number of meetings and documentation. The CPA key worker will need to identify all contributors to the care plan and involve these in an effective way, including John's attendance at the planning meeting (with his agreement). The likely membership may be extensive and will include:

- John Boucher
- CPN/CPA key worker
- social worker
- consultant psychiatrist
- occupational therapist/day service worker
- general practitioner.

The client may have reservations about attending the meeting with so many people present and the CPA key worker needs to check out what will be acceptable. Where people are not to be invited or cannot attend, their views can be elicited, inputs clarified and copies of the completed care plan provided for them. Also relevant are the concerns of others who may not always be contributing directly to the care plan. In this case, this would include representatives of the housing department and possibly the residential care staff where John's mother resides.

For the CPA plan to be effective, the desired outcomes need to be stated and the inputs of all contributors clarified and recorded through the care plan. This may require negotiation and the use of lateral or collegiate authority where the CPA key worker has no legitimate or structural control over colleagues whose commitment needs to be ensured. The CPA key worker may be required to provide a leadership role which may involve more assertive behaviour than hitherto displayed. This will include chairing a meeting effectively.

Utilizing and coordinating available resources, contributing to service planning

Successful completion of the CPA key worker's role requires a shift from focusing only in one's own input to mobilizing a wide range of resources. Therefore, the CPN needs to be aware of what resources are available which John can make use of. His needs may not be met entirely by people working within the mental health-care system. For example, he may benefit from attending the adult education centre. The needs assessment approach built into the CPA process involves the identification of resource deficits. In theory, the deficits identified within individual care plans can be aggregated, fed into the service development process and so inform the business and strategic planning of health and social service authorities.

However, in practice this can be problematic. Many health-care workers have difficulty in adopting a needs-led rather than a resource-led approach. This means that clients get what is available instead of what they need. This can lead to conservatism and inertia within services. At the same time many workers have become acclimatized to 'complaining' about inadequate resource levels. This behaviour has to an extent become embedded in the culture and may be caused by concerns that if resource levels are inadequate, reductions may be imposed. In other words, it is necessary to say that there is not enough to go around to ensure maintenance of existing funding levels. However, the failure to identify resource deficits within individual care plans contradict this claim. A mind shift is required from practitioners and a willingness to engage in the business planning cycle, an area traditionally regarded as the domain of managers.

Organization of self and others; priority setting

Being an effective CPA key worker will involve a high degree of personal organization. Time is needed to organize meetings and to prepare and distribute care plans. Ensuring the involvement and commitment of others is not always straightforward. Increasingly, more time is needed for the organization of effective care and this is not always recognized by clinical staff as legitimate and credible and this trend is enforced by service contracts that define activity only in terms of direct client contact.

The CPA key worker will need to ensure the availability of the other contributors to the care plan. It cannot be assumed that people will be available to attend meetings. Some teams will find it convenient to schedule regular clinical slots for CPA planning and reviews which will make the coordination of meetings easier to achieve. Good administrative support and systems are necessary to make the CPA effective.

Patients such as John Boucher should be regarded as a priority. The CPA plan should define a frequency of contact with him and outline contingency arrangements in the event of loss of contact. For the CPA key worker sufficient time needs to be set aside to allow for not just the direct contact but also for the inevitable planning and liaison work involved. A number of services are being reconfigured to allow appropriate targeting of this client group.

Recognizing training needs

It should not be assumed that all mental health nurses have the necessary skills to act as a CPA key worker. Many services will expect nurses employed at a particular level of seniority to undertake this role. A degree of honesty is necessary between the nurse who does not feel confident or competent to carry out the considerable tasks described and her manager. The underimplementation of the CPA may be directly attributable to skills, knowledge and experience deficits in those staff designated as CPA key workers. Defining the competencies and knowledge necessary is the responsibility of both clinicians and managers and training programmes and opportunities need to be developed accordingly.

Using clinical supervision

Finally, as with all aspects of mental health nursing practice, the relationship of clinical supervision to practice should be discussed. The extent and effectiveness of clinical supervision will vary from service to service. Some areas will have introduced systems to identify priority clients for consideration in supervision. Where this is not in place individual practitioners are recommended to use supervision to review the care being provided for clients such as John Boucher on a routine basis. Clinical supervision can be an effective forum for exploring any difficulties in implementing the care plan and in particular some of the complexities involved in mobilizing other professionals.

RECONFIGURING COMMUNITY MENTAL HEALTH TEAMS: AN EXAMPLE

Introduction: purpose of the study

This section demonstrates the practical application of a number of management processes within a community mental health service. It attempts to illustrate the relationship between management theory and practice and describes how a manager can act as a change agent to bring about improvements in services. A brief overview of the national and local service context is provided. The reasons for change and the necessary processes involved are defined. Some models of change management are proposed. The study describes the 'reconfiguration' of two community mental health teams (CMHTs) and a psychiatric day hospital. The project involved changes to structure of teams and how priorities were determined and required significant adjustments to the content of some individuals' work. We provide an example of how managers must understand the impact of political and policy pressures in the wider environment and also the complexities of multidisciplinary working. Additionally, the need to maintain the service whilst making significant changes is described.

Some descriptions of change within organizations recount how there was darkness, chaos, high labour cost and then came the manager with his or her change plan and then there was light, efficiency, low unit cost and widespread happiness! The temptation to describe such heroism has been resisted here. In practice, bringing about change generally relies on those initiating and implementing it having patience and sensitivity, keeping focused on what they need to do and recognizing and capitalizing on opportunities when they present themselves. Nevertheless, change theories provide a necessary structure without which little of lasting benefit will be achieved and widespread alienation could result. Hopefully, this section will give clinicians and managers some ideas about what can be done to modernize services and how to go about it.

The following processes are illustrated:

- planning and managing changes in mental health services
- using existing resources more effectively – targeting and reconfiguration
- identifying and responding to demands in the wider environment
- use of CPA tiering as means of categorizing workload
- integration of service elements and avoidance of duplication
- negotiation and persuasion to help people change
- promoting role clarity.

Broad policy context

The multidisciplinary CMHT has become part of the mental health service landscape over the past 15 years. Much studied and criticized (Galvin and McCarthy 1994, Onyett and Ford 1996, Patmore and Weaver 1991), it remains the most common model of community service delivery. Widespread variations in size, composition and location of bases and operational methods have been found. Significant complications have been observed about the management arrangements for these teams. Typical team membership comprises a consultant psychiatrist, community psychiatric nurses (CPNs), occupational therapist (OT), psychologist, social workers and administrative staff. Poor or non-existent identification of priorities and interprofessional conflict were typical problems observed. Despite this critique, the CMHT remains the most common service model used to deliver community mental health services to a locality. Recently, there have been examples of teams being developed or restructured from existing staff groups to ensure appropriate targeting of people with severe and enduring mental illnesses (White *et al.* 1996).

Local policy context

The locality services comprised two CMHTs and a day hospital serving the population aged 16–65 in two adjacent towns. The service had built up around the psychiatric day hospital which had opened some 15 years earlier. It had been the only element of community mental health service in the locality, with inpatient treatment provided at a large Victorian hospital in the neighbouring health authority. This was scheduled for closure within the next decade. The day hospital became a base for CPNs and social workers and there was some progressive growth in staff members with the addition of psychology and TO staff. This formed the origins of community mental health team A. Additionally, by the late 1980s a range of informal social day care had been developed by social services. A community mental health centre accommodating a small team (team D) in the neighbouring town was opened in 1992.

The overall membership of the teams and day hospital included consultant psychiatrists, nurses (CPNs and day hospital nurses), OTs, psychologists and administrative and ancillary staff. Some variations to working practices had developed with team A members accepting and responding to direct referrals from GPs whilst team B pooled and allocated referrals in a weekly meeting. The day hospital was a 'tertiary' service with no direct GP referrals being accepted.

In 1990 its purpose was defined as providing a level of treatment and support not available within the CMHTs for patients not needing or not wanting hospital admission. Ostensibly a range of services was available to meet different levels of need and dependency. The day hospital provided a range of time-limited/topic-based therapeutic groups (e.g. anxiety management, assertiveness training) to which members of the CMHT could refer. Patients requiring long-term help from the day hospital team would need to be referred to and accepted by either of the psychiatrists.

The locality manager with a mental health nursing background had overall responsibility for the effective delivery of services and held line management responsibility for nursing and administrative staff. Other staff groups retained their own professional management structures. Such management arrangements are by no means untypical in CMHTs and had been repeatedly criticized within the trust. Many had argued unsuccessfully for a more linear arrangement with all staff reporting to a locality manager. This was resisted by senior psychologists and occupational therapists, many of whom felt strongly that professional management was essential. A consequence of these complex arrangements was that the locality manager had to liaise effectively with other managers to ensure the effective operation and integration of the service. Moreover, any proposed changes to policy and service developments involved extensive negotiation. Potentially the scope for intergroup conflict and divergent goals was high (Zagier Roberts 1994). In practice, the various managers responsible for the locality services did not see the complex management arrangements as an obstacle to change. However, this was dependent upon the individuals achieving good collaborative relationships rather than the structural arrangements.

Change models

It is not the intention here to provide the reader with a wide theoretical overview of change management. This is available elsewhere in the extensive literature available about planning and managing change (e.g. Clarke 1994). Nevertheless, it would be unwise to attempt change without having grasped basic principles about process, style and obstacles, so a summary of key tenets is provided.

First, a word of warning. Change programmes should not be embarked upon lightly. Resistance is almost inevitable and there will always be winner and losers as (Clarke 1994), Machiavelli warned 'There is nothing more difficult to plan, more doubtful of success, nor more dangerous to manage than the creation of a new system. For the initiator has the enmity of all who would profit by the preservation of the old institutions, and merely lukewarm defenders in those who should gain by the new ones'. Furthermore, it would be foolish to regard resistance as merely resistance – some of it may be founded upon previous experience of failed change programmes. Staff in the health and social services have undergone continual changes to structure, systems and processes and so may be suffering from change fatigue.

Make sure that the change is necessary and plan very carefully. Changes within commercial organizations are generally driven by market factors and fears of loss of business. The NHS was subject to market forces in the same way until the creation of the internal market legislated in the NHS and Community Care Act 1990. This introduced a more commercial orientation within the service and an adoption of management and business processes. Greater attention has been paid to the threat and impact of 'external demands' (Beckhard and Harris 1987) which may necessitate change. This notion of external demand draws upon the analogy of an organization or service being like an organism which needs to adapt to its environment to survive.

Many of the approaches to change management rely upon the themes of identification and analysis of problems with the present situation and the development of a change plan, its implementation and evaluation. An enduring model has been that of Lewin (1951) who defined three basic steps:

- unfreezing the current situation
- leading to moving
- refreezing – setting a new equilibrium.

Unfreezing is concerned with creating the climate for change and takes place when the motivation for some form of change occurs. This may arise from a number of possible reasons including: lack of confirmation or disconfirmation because expectations have not been met; induction of guilt or anxiety due to some action or inaction; and psychological safety when a former obstacle to change has been removed. *Moving* is concerned with mobilizing energy and resources towards the desired aim, the new situation. It includes the action phase of the change process. *Refreezing* is achieved when the change is integrated into the system and stabilized into a new equilibrium. Kurt Lewin (1951) developed the concept of force field analysis where driving forces for change are identified as well as restraining forces opposing change. Beckhard and Harris (1987) have advocated an accurate definition of the change problem and a definition of the features of the present state which have to change in order to reach the desired future state. Similarly, another researcher has proposed three basic questions for consideration:

- What kind of future do we want to have?
- What is our present state in relation to moving to that future?
- What can be done to progress from the present state to that future?

Bennis *et al.* (1985) put forward three change strategies: power coercive, normative re-educative, and rational empirical. The power coercive strategy relies on power, authority and influence to ensure compliance with change. People are simply instructed to do things differently. This approach may be effective in extreme conditions and where resistance can be dealt with easily. However, change may not be integrated into the value system and people may revert to previous behaviour when not closely supervised. The *normative re-educative* strategy assumes that attitudes change through personal growth and development. This approach may be seen as 'bottom up' and is based upon the belief that people need to be involved in all aspects of the changes which affect them. It is suggested that this approach is more likely to promote more effective long-term change and greater levels of ownership of the new system. The *rational empirical* approach assumes that people are rational beings, motivated by self-interest, who will follow reason and make sensible decisions based on sound knowledge of the given situation. Although it may be viewed as a top-down approach, it is nevertheless often seen as desirable and beneficial. Our experience indicates that wise change agents do not 'put all their eggs in any one basket' but utilize a combination of approaches depending on the given context and nature of the situation.

The reconfiguration project

The approach adopted relied upon the following steps:

- identification of external demands
- analysis of present state
- specifying the desired future state
- defining change tasks
- implementation and evaluation.

Identification of external demands

The locality services had developed in an incremental way with resources in the community generally increasing as the neighbouring mental hospital was run down. However, this growth and development had been service or resource led rather than needs led. It was not possible to predict the impact of the NHS and Community Care Act, particularly care management, the advent of GP fundholding and then the increasingly explicit requirement to target services upon people with severe and enduring mental illnesses that emerged during the early 1990s. The changing and apparently irreconcilable demands made it difficult to continue delivering the service in the present way.

During a series of meetings staff in the various teams were encouraged to express their views about the strengths and weaknesses of the present service and its readiness to cope with the changing demands. A number of local and national pressures were identified.

- Fewer inpatient beds (more patients with chronic difficulties living in the community).
- Expectations of GPs rising – too many referrals, some inappropriate.
- People with serious mental illness, identified as priority group by the Department of Health, were getting squeezed.
- Growing media criticism of the safety of community mental health care policy, leading to risk-averse climate.
- Requirement to fully implement the CPA, Section (117) of the 1983 Mental Health Act, supervision register and supervised discharge.
- Need to integrate care management and CPA.

- No new mental health strategy from health purchaser for three years.
- Limited growth and drive to cost containment.
- Need to deliver contracted activity.
- Patient's Charter/Mental Health Patient's Charter standards.

Simultaneously strengths of the service were appraised and its readiness to adapt.

- A core of experienced and well-qualified staff.
- Good facilities.
- Open climate in which to discuss and address issues.
- Managers and senior clinical staff working well together.
- Local autonomy to effect change.

Analysing the present state

An accurate enough view of why the present situation needs to change is required. This needs to take account of the whole service system rather than concentrate on one component alone. Additionally, this needs to be a shared perspective and be widely communicated to and understood by all staff. Given some of the difficulties in implementing change and low potential benefits, it is essential to achieve a wide recognition of the need to change before attempting anything.

Lack of space here prevents a full description of the situation but some aspects are provided as examples. Overall, the present structure and operation of the locality services were poorly equipped to deal with these changes in the external world. The high levels of access to the service enjoyed by GPs had meant that the priority patients with severe and enduring illnesses were getting a residual level of service. No eligibility criteria had been set to determine who should receive the service and so existing resources were continually being stretched to meet growing demand. The generic roles undertaken by CPNs and OTs did not allow sufficient targeting of the priority groups or the development and concentration of skills needed to look after them. This contrasted with the clearer position of the Social Services department which had introduced eligibility criteria to allow targeting of people with severe and enduring illnesses. The policy imperatives of fully implementing the CPA, Section (117), supervised discharge and the supervision register could not be achieved under the present condition.

A growing emphasis on performance management had led to a climate where measuring those things that can be measured was increasingly important. For the day hospital there had been an expectation to deliver a volume of services rather than a more individually focused service. The success of the service was determined by how many people were attending each day. This has been described as the 'bums on seats' approach. This emphasis on volume meant that staff had to treat patients in large groups which could not cater for variations in the clients' levels of disability and motivation. Being the only available service, it had historically been required to provide a range of services, including a type of general support which was now defined as social care (DoH 1989). The Social Services department had developed a number of social care services which were more appropriate for a number of people attending the day hospital. On one hand the day hospital risked becoming an obsolete service but on the other this presented an opportunity for some patients to move to more appropriate services, thereby reducing duplication and releasing time for the team.

The introduction of the CPA in 1991 was partially successful in achieving multidisciplinary care planning but its coverage was incomplete owing to initially being largely restricted to patients subject to Section (117). Later and clearer guidance from the DoH had indicated a tiered approach to the CPA and prescribed a wide coverage (DoH 1996a). There had been resistance and even hostility to the CPA in some quarters, with many regarding it as a bureaucratic exercise and merely formalizing what was being done already. Within the locality services there had been a recognition that the CPA could not only help to increase the care inputs but improve coordination and communication between those contributing to the care plan. However, this was time consuming and probably not compatible with the generic roles being undertaken by the CPNs and OTs. It would require some shift from direct clinical activity with a high emphasis on volume to more indirect work organizing care inputs which would reduce present activity levels. Different skills were required to carry out the CPA effectively so it made sense for a smaller group of staff to concentrate on doing this properly rather than spreading it thinly. A strong culture had developed which valued 'doing the business' with accompanying expectations about high volumes of activity and responsiveness to GPs.

The Social Services department introduced a care management system in 1994 with accompanying eligibility criteria which targeted those service users with more enduring mental health problems. The introduction of eligibility criteria effectively restricted the type of clients that social workers accepted. This shortfall would have to be met by the trust's staff, thereby increasing workload. On the plus side, an agreement had been reached with the Social Services authority that social workers would act as CPA workers. This approach was based upon a recognition of a similarity between the aims of the CPA and care management.

Finally, there was uncertainty about who should initiate any change. In theory the NHS trusts are service organizations providing specified service for the purchaser. The purchasing health authority was tasked with preparing a mental health strategy which should provide a blueprint for services. This was some years off and waiting for the new strategy was not an available option.

To summarize, a number of potent external demands or drivers (Clarke 1994) had emerged. The local services had developed in an incremental way, were overextended and poorly targeted and were no longer sustainable in their present format. There was some support for reconfiguring the service to try and address the new demands.

Defining the future state
Through a series of meetings all staff members were encouraged to think about ways in which the demands described could be met and how the revamped

service might look. This has been referred to as 'defining the future state'. The importance of this is to move from a hazy idea that something needs to be done towards defining a more concrete and realizable project. This will not only reduce uncertainty and expose different assumptions that individuals may hold about the process but also enables identification of the necessary action steps to achieve this future state. As no increase in funding could be relied upon, the project would have to use existing resources in a different way. This has been described as reconfiguration.

Examples of the desired future state would be to ensure that every patient with a severe and enduring illness would be identified and assigned a CPA key worker who would organize and ensure the implementation of a multidisciplinary care plan. A further example would be the establishment of a referral meeting for the CPNs in team A in order to ensure the appropriateness of referrals. Additionally, an urgent assessment clinic was set up to deal with more urgent referrals that could not wait for the allocation meeting. This enabled a more systematic approach to managing the workload. Paradoxically the high level of exposure and responsiveness to GPs had meant diaries were full and CPNs found it difficult to respond to urgent referrals. Yet another example would be the introduction of a screening system whereby a CPN and social worker would visit the inpatient unit each week to ascertain which patients would need care management of former (multidisciplinary) CPA.

It was also necessary to think about ways in which the service might operate in the longer term but which were not realizable in the short term. Developing a shared perspective of how things might be but recognizing why this cannot be achieved is important. Obstacles would include lack of agency agreement between the trust and Social Services preventing fuller integration of CPA with care management and the lack of knowledge about the content of the forthcoming mental health strategy document from the purchaser. Local staff would have only minimal influence over these factors so to an extent would be second guessing.

Defining the change tasks

The development of two teams working with a differentiated clientele was the most logical model of service. Certain staff would work exclusively with patients meeting the criteria for CPA levels two and three, those clients with severe and enduring illnesses. This would ensure more effective targeting for the severe and enduring clientele and the scope to develop more specific programmes to meet individual needs. This could be described as a functional structure where staff would carry out different roles according to the client need.

There is an old story about a person asking for directions being told 'I would not start from here!'. If these services were being commissioned now, the structure would be very different. However, it was not possible to close down, reorganize and start again. It was necessary to maintain the service or 'keep the shop open'. Moreover, some of the changes would inevitably need to be evolutionary but should not become so protracted as to lose momentum. A number of action steps or change tasks were identified. These would involve using the day hospital staff as the core of a team dedicated to the severe and enduring client population. Some of the activity currently undertaken by this team for the CPA level one clientele would need to be carried out by others. The existing day hospital team would not be sufficient to look after all of these clients and looked certain to require supplementing by the redeployment of CPN time.

It was necessary to identify as accurately as possible the total workload of the teams, who was working with which clients and what the impact upon workload would be of changing the composition of the caseloads. It had emerged that there was some duplication in that the clients attending the day hospital had CPA key workers who were CPNs from the CMHT. There was scope to streamline things by ensuring that as far as possible the CPA key worker was the person who had the most direct contact with the client. The following was agreed.

- Reconfiguring the service – so that clients are targeted according to their needs by staff undertaking more specified roles.
- Establishing and maintaining a locality CPA register.
- Changes were necessary to CPN roles. Across the locality a total of three people would need to work exclusively with the severe and enduring population. Ideally people would change their role on a voluntary basis.
- No new referrals of level one CPA clients should be accepted by the day hospital.
- Some of the topic-based groups for level one CPA clients, e.g. anxiety and management, previously undertaken by the day hospital team would need to be carried out by the CPNs in team A.
- Keeping morale 'good enough' and promoting commitment.

Implementation so far

It was necessary to gauge how people viewed the change project. Team meetings and individual supervision sessions were used for this. There were some supporters for the proposals, some were neutral and some in opposition. It was necessary to identify and build upon a critical mass (Clarke 1994) of support for the changes. It was also necessary to appraise the strength and validity of any resistance. Defining the future state by means of a draft operational policy helped people to focus on what the service could look like. Meetings were convened for the wider stakeholding group including staff from Social Services and the independent sector. Staff likely to be most affected were encouraged to visit other services where similar changes had been attempted and to report back. A common cause of resistance occurs when people fear that they will have no role in the future. Maximum opportunities were taken to communicate formally and informally about the proposals. Insufficient communication about changes can be a common cause of failure to implement change effectively.

Following extensive negotiation and discussion of the merits of the change one generic CPN in each team agreed to work exclusively with CPA level two and three clients and a staff nurse vacancy was upgraded temporarily to create a third CPN post to work exclusively with this clientele. OT and nursing roles in the day hospital were similarly adjusted. No new level two and three clients were accepted by the generic CPNs and existing clients in those categories were gradually transferred to the newly established team.

CPNs accepting new work were redesigned as 'the intake team' and were able to maintain initiatives such as an urgent assessment clinic and have begun to provide topic-focused therapeutic groups for clients previously referred to the day hospital. Staff in the level two and three team were able to consolidate relationships with social workers and have begun the screening initiative with inpatients to identify clients eligible for complex CPA care management at an early stage.

Evaluation

No formal evaluation has taken place of the reconfiguration project but there are some indications that the level two and three clients are more engaged in the service and that identification of this clientele has been more effective. The screening initiative has improved identification of those clients in the care management/formal CPA category and has allowed speedier appointment of a CPA key worker. Nursing and occupational therapy roles have changed in the manner planned. The CPA register has been set up and maintained and accurate information is available about collective and individual caseloads. Working relationships between the trust staff and Social Services/voluntary sector have strengthened as the overall number of staff involved with this client group have reduced.

To date, the reconfiguration project has not required anyone to change their role unwillingly. Justifiable anxieties were expressed about the break-up of some existing working relationships and any professional consequences of moving away from generic roles. It was thought that working exclusively with clients experiencing long-term mental health problems would be stressful and lower job satisfaction. However, these concerns have been more than offset by achieving greater role clarity for staff working in both groups. Average caseload size has actually reduced for both groups of CPNs.

On the negative side one of the more difficult areas has been the replacement of the range of topic-based groups for the level one clients. This is currently under examination. Some argue that there is now a positive bias towards those clients in the CPA level two and three tiers. This may be a justified criticism but it may have been a necessary stage to work through in order to arrive at an equitable distribution of services and to demonstrate how much of the available resource is required to look after this population.

CONCLUSION

This chapter began by placing the role of the mental health nurse as manager in a historical context. A discussion of selected key issues and concepts of management followed. In addition, we discussed key issues relating to current aspects of mental health legislation including the 1983 Mental Health Act and the planned review, the Care Programme Approach, care management, supervision registers and the 1995 Mental Health (Patients in the Community) Act. Two examples were then presented to illustrate the application of these concepts to the everyday work of mental health nurses working in managerial capacities at different levels.

Finally, one of the authors (MAE) would like to share with readers the following experience by way of reflecting on the role of the mental health nurse. In a memorial lecture to the late Eileen Skellern who was an innovative matron at the Maudsley Hospital, Professor Annie Altschul, the first Professor in Psychiatric Nursing in this country, declared:

> *People ask me what makes a good psychiatric nurse? I tell them, I do not know, that is, I do not know how to describe her, but when I see a good one in action I can tell. It is just like a good piece of music, I know one when I hear it but I cannot tell you what notes go into making it or exactly how it was put together!*

This may be seen as far too romantic a view and even too good to be true. Indeed, Professor Jennifer Wilson-Barnett of King's College, London, said as much the following year when she was giving the same memorial lecture. Professor Wilson-Barnett argued instead for a more scientific approach quantifying and measuring what the nurse's role is and what it should be concerned with, etc.

Professor Altschul had inspired many psychiatric nurses, including the author, and Professor Wilson-Barnett was his teacher. Both remain shining lights in the world of nursing. In conclusion, however, we would like to suggest that successful mental health nurse managers have not only developed the art of playing good music but can also deftly turn their hands to occasionally conducting the odd piece.

REFERENCES

Barker, P. (1998) Advancing practice in mental health nursing: developing the core. In: Rolfe, G. and Fulbrook, P. (eds) *Advanced Nursing Practice*. Butterworth-Heinemann, Oxford.

Bennis, W., Benne, K., Chin, R. *et al.* (eds) (1985) *The Planning of Change*, 4th edn. Holt, Rhinehart and Winston, London.

Blanchard, K. and Johnson, S. (1983) *The One Minute Manager*. Berkley Books, New York.

Carpenter, J. and Sbaraini, S. (1996) Involving service users and carers in the care programme approach. *Journal of Mental Health*, 5(5): pp. 483–488.

Clarke, J. (1994) *Managing Social Policy*. Sage Publications.

DoH (1989) *Caring for People: community care in the next decade and beyond, caring for the 1990s*. HMSO, London.

DoH (1991a) *Care Management and Assessment: practitioners' guide*. HMSO, London.

DoH (1991b) *Care Management and Assessment: managers' guide*. HMSO, London.

DoH and Welsh Office (1993) *Code of Practice: Mental Health Act 1983*. HMSO, London.

DoH (1994) *Working in Partnership: a collaborative approach to care. Report of the Mental Health Nursing Review Team*. HMSO, London.

DoH (1996a) *An Audit Pack for Monitoring the Care Programme Approach*. NHS Executive, London.

DoH (1996b) *Building Bridges: a guide to arrangements for interagency working for the care and protection of severely mentally ill people*. HMSO, London.

DoH (1998) *Modernising Mental Health Services: safe, sound and supportive*. HMSO, London.

Ford, R. *et al.* (1996) Does intensive case management work? Clinical, social and quality of life outcomes from a controlled study, *Journal of Mental Health*, 5(4): pp. 361–368.

Forrest, I. (1983) Management education and training of nurses: research study. *Journal of Advanced Nursing* 8: 139–145.

Forsyth, P. (1994) *First Things First: how to manage your time for maximum performance*. Pitman, London.

Galvin, S.W. and McCarthy, S. (1994) Multi-disciplinary community teams: clinging to the wreckage. *Journal of Mental Health* 3: 157–166.

Griffiths, R. (1988) *Community Care: Agenda for Action. A report to the Secretary of State for Social Services*, HMSO.

Handy, C. (1985) *Understanding Organisations*. Pelican Books, London.

Hersey, P. and Blanchard, K.H. (1982) *Management of organization behaviour* 4th edn. Prentice-Hall. Englewood Cliffs, NJ.

HMSO (1990) *National Health Service and Community Care Act 1990*, HMSO.

House, R.J. (1988) Leadership research: some forgotten, ignored or overlooked findings. In: Hunt H.G., Baliga, B.R., Dachler, H.P. and Shriesheim, C.A. (eds) *Emerging Leadership Vistas*. Lexington, Boston.

House of Commons (1994) *Better Off in the Community? The care of people who are seriously mentally ill. Health Committee, First Report, Session 1993–94*. HMSO.

Hudson, B. (1992) Mental health Policy in England in the 1990s: Which way for the care programme approach? Short Reports, *Journal of Health Service Management*.

Hunt, G. (1994) *Expanding the role of the nurse: the scope of professional practice*. Blackwell Scientific Press.

Johns, C. and Graham J. (1994) Using a reflection model of nursing. *Nursing Standard*, 11 (2): 34–8.

Kane, R. *et al.* (1991) What cost case management in long term care? *Social Services Review* June, HMSO.

King's Fund (1981) *The Preparation of Senior Nurse Managers in the NHS: a report of peer group exchange seminars 1977–80*. King's Fund Centre, London.

Koontz, H. and Weihrich, H. (1988) *Management*. McGraw Hill.

Lewin, K. (1951) *Field Theory in Social Science*. Harper and Row, New York.

MacGregor, D. (1960) *The Human Side of Enterprise*. McGraw Hill, New York.

Marelli, T.M. (1993) *Nurse Manager's Survival Guide: practical answers to everyday problems*. Mosby, St Louis.

Masterton, A. (1997) *Getting Results with Time Management*. Library Association Publishing, London.

Ministry of Health and Scottish Home and Health Department (1966) *Report of the Committee on Senior Nursing Staff Structure (Salmon Report)*. HMSO, London.

Mintzberg, H. (1973) *The Nature of Managerial Work*. Harper and Row, New York.

North, C., Ritchie, J. and Ward, K. (1993) *Factors Influencing the Implementation of The Care Programme Approach – A research study carried out for the DoH by Social and Community Planning Research*, HMSO.

Onyett, S. and Ford, R. (1996) Multi-disciplinary community team: where is the wreckage? *Journal of Mental Health* 5: 47–55.

Ouchi, W.G. (1981) *Theory Z: how American business can meet the Japanese challenge*. Addison-Wesley, Reading, MA.

Patmore, C. and Weaver, T. (1991) *Community Mental Health Issues: lessons for planners and managers*. GPMH, London.

Peters, T. (1988) *Thriving in chaos*. London. MacMillan.

Ritchie, J. *et al.* (1994) *The report of the inquiry into the care and treatment of Christopher Clunis*. HMSO

Rocchiccioli, J.T. and Tilbury, M.S. (1998) *Clinical Leadership in Nursing*. W.B. Saunders, Philadelphia.

Rogers, A., Pilgrim, D. and Lacey, R. (1993) *Experiencing Psychiatry: users' views of services*. Macmillan, London.

Rowden, R. (1987) Training for management. *Journal of Clinical Practice Education and Management* 3: 579–580.

Ryan, T. and Hardy, L. (1996) Mental Health Legislation: A time to act? *Care Plan*, 3(2) pp. 22–25.

Schein, E.H. (1984) Organisation culture and leadership. In: Coming to a new awareness of organisational culture, *Sloan Management Review*, Winter.

Social Services Select Committee (1985) *Community Care with Special References to Adult Mentally Ill and Mentally Handicapped People*. HMSO, London.

Social Services Select Committee (1990) *Community care: Services for people with a mental handicap and people with a mental illness*. HMSO, London.

Tetrault, L.A., Schriesheim, C.A. and Neider, L.L. (1988) Leadership training interventions: a review. *Developing Leadership Excellence: Journal of Management Development (Special Issue)* 7(15): 10–20.

Vroom, V.H. and Deci, E.L. (eds) (1974) *Management and Motivation*, p. 367. Penguin, Harmondsworth.

Vroom, V. and Vetton (1973) *Leadership and Decision Making*. University of Pittsburgh Press, Pittsburgh.

Watkins, M. *et al.* (Eds) (1996) *Collaborative Community Mental Health Care*, Arnold.

White, K.M. (1998) Planned change. In: Rocchiccioli, J.T. and Tilbury, M.S. (Eds) *Clinical Leadership in Nursing*. W.B. Saunder, Philadelphia.

White, K., Ness, M., Crissy, T. and McNamee, G. (1996) Makey Community Bureau Mental Health Resources work, *Psychiatric Bulletin* 20: 93–96.

Wright, S.G. (1993) Management as an integral part of nursing. *Journal of Nursing Management* 1: 129–132.

Zagier Roberts, V. (1994) *The Unconcious at Work*. Routledge, London.

7 THE NURSE AS SUPERVISOR

Norman MacDonald

OBJECTIVES

After reading this chapter, you should be able to:

- define clinical supervision
- demonstrate an understanding of the functions of clinical supervision
- show an increased awareness of the relevance and importance of clinical supervision in mental health nursing
- show an increased awareness of the issues relating to the organization and implementation of supervision and the relevant skills.

INTRODUCTION

Clinical supervision is essentially a working alliance between a supervisor – most commonly a manager or professional with more clinical experience – and a worker or group of workers. It helps workers to reflect on themselves in the working situation by giving an account of the work undertaken and receiving feedback, guidance and appraisal as appropriate.

For some years there has been a move towards ensuring that clinical supervision is available for all nursing staff working in clinical areas. The interpretation of what is required, and the degree to which it has been implemented, seems to have varied greatly from one area to another. It has long been a process associated with psychotherapy and counselling practice and in a quite different sense has been a statutory requirement for midwives.

The relevance of the process of clinical supervision to mental health nursing is clear, where much work is based on developing a relationship with people in distress, which can be frustrating or itself distressing. Certain procedures, for example administration of medication or completion of documentation, are amenable simply to being observed by another member of staff to ensure that the work is being properly undertaken. However, issues relating to the development of therapeutic relationships are self-evidently more complex and a different approach is required. The importance of clinical supervision will be considered first in the broadest sense and the specific issues relating to mental health nursing will then be addressed in more detail.

There has been great enthusiasm from the government and statutory bodies alike for the implementation of clinical supervision throughout the nursing profession. The UKCC underlined its commitment with six key statements designed to 'assist the development and establishment of effective supervision' (UKCC 1996).

- Clinical supervision supports practice, enabling practitioners to *maintain and promote standards of care*.
- Clinical supervision is a *practice-focused professional relationship* involving a practitioner reflecting on practice guided by a skilled supervisor.
- The process of clinical supervision should be developed by practitioners and managers according to local circumstances. Ground rules should be agreed so that practitioners and supervisors approach supervision openly and confidently and are aware of what is involved.
- Every practitioner should have *access* to clinical supervision. Each supervisor should supervise a realistic number of practitioners.
- *Preparation* for supervisors can be effected using 'in-house' or external education programmes. The principles and relevance of clinical supervision should be included in pre- and postregistration education programmes.
- *Evaluation* of clinical supervision is needed to assess how it influences care, practice standards and the service. Evaluation systems should be determined locally.

If, then, it is clearly relevant at a clinical level and encouraged at a policy level, it is perhaps strange that the implementation of clinical supervision has not been a universal happening, never mind a success. It is worth considering why this is the case and in order to do this, the various aspects and functions of clinical supervision will be explored and the specific problems associated with its implementation will be addressed. Strategies for effective supervision at organizational, clinical and personal levels will then be suggested. This is too important an issue to be ignored and clinical supervision will not implement itself.

Mental health nurses work at different levels in a wide range of settings using different approaches with a wide range of people, including patients, clients, residents, colleagues, students and relatives. For the sake of consistency and simplicity, irrespective of setting, context or relationship, the terms 'nurse' and 'client' will be used. Equally, the nurse will be referred to as 'she' simply for linguistic convenience – no gender issues are intended to be raised. The rich variation in work must not, however, be forgotten.

There has been a range of perspectives on clinical supervision but certain key issues consistently emerge, primarily:

- the maintenance of quality of work and protection of the client
- helping the nurse develop knowledge, skills and attitudes in the context of a trusting and supportive relationship
- supporting the nurse working in difficult and demanding situations, often in a climate of change.

These key themes have been categorized as

- *normative* – acknowledging that the supervisor/manager has a duty to ensure the highest standards of care

- *formative* – developing the nurses' skills, understanding and competence
- *restorative* – supporting the nurse in the light of the stressful and emotional component of their professional work (Proctor, in Marken and Payne 1986).

One other possible dimension of the process of clinical supervision is the development of self-awareness. This is the exploration of the nurse's feelings and how those feelings relate to her behaviour in the clinical area (Barber and Norman 1987). The importance of this aspect of clinical supervision was acknowledged by the NHSME (1993) when it stated that it was '... central to the process of learning and to the expansion of the scope of practice, and should be seen as a method of encouraging self-assessment and analytical and reflective skills'. Specifically relating to mental health nursing, Scanlon & Weir note that it is 'essential to be aware of psychological boundaries. It would be easy to get drawn into someone else's psychopathology, and supervision is an essential safeguard' (Scanlon and Weir 1997, p. 298).

There are clear similarities between reflective practice, self-awareness and clinical supervision. It may be argued that the first two are simply structured ways of individual analytical thinking, while the third relies on a second person – the supervisor. This has clear implications for resources. If the nurse can simply take a few minutes to write or think how she might have behaved and felt towards clients, this is obviously less expensive than taking up the time of two professionals undertaking clinical supervision. However, Casement (1985) has argued that the development of what he referred to as an 'inner supervisor' could only take place and be maintained with a background of working with a skilled supervisor. This is consistent with Luft and Inghams (Luft 1984) who suggest, with their graphic Johari Window, that in order to develop self-awareness we need to address issues that are apparent to others but not to ourselves. At a very basic level, sometimes we are unable to see the wood for the trees and other perspectives are necessary. Casement's 'inner supervisor' could not therefore convincingly perform the formative or restorative functions of clinical supervision, let alone the normative.

In 1994 the Clothier Report (DoH 1994) identified wide-ranging implications from the series of failures to monitor the circumstances and work of Beverley Allitt, who was infamously responsible for the deaths of a number of children under her care. It is not surprising that the report raised the importance of the normative aspect of supervision – monitoring quality of care and ensuring the safety of the patient. To a great extent the debate on clinical supervision has moved away from the more analytic models based on psychotherapy so that it now focuses on this normative aspect. This is of course at the expense of the more developmental formative and restorative aspects, where the skills and feelings of the nurse are central.

The focus on the normative aspect of supervision would not of itself be a problem were it not for the fact that this may not be totally compatible with the other two aspects being implemented, particularly in terms of whether there is a direct link between the supervision and management issues (Bishop 1994). To illustrate this, consideration will now be given to each of the three aspects in turn, in terms of organization, administration and focus.

NORMATIVE SUPERVISION: ISSUES OF QUALITY OF CARE AND CLIENT SAFETY

As with each aspect of clinical supervision, work can be undertaken on a formal or informal basis. A formal approach would involve regular planned meetings in work time. The agenda would be set with a view to monitoring standards, auditing aspects of care and evaluating specific areas of work. These areas might range from caseload management or role in the team to more personal issues such as time management or record keeping, perhaps even issues like the level of sickness or timekeeping. The supervisor would typically be a line manager, who could dictate the agenda in an authoritative way, the main goal being to enhance the organization (Driscoll 1996). There are clear similarities between this and a formal appraisal scheme. One study found concern that such a process might be used to identify faults, which may subsequently be referred to as evidence in disciplinary procedures (McCallion and Baxter 1995).

An informal approach with a focus on the normative aspect of clinical supervision might involve a response to a crisis or to a particular difficulty or issue in the clinical area. This might range from looking at how a particular incident of violence was handled or might have been prevented to addressing gossip or conflicts within the team. The work could be instigated by either the manager or the supervisee, but typically probably the former.

It would be ridiculous to argue that there should not be any monitoring of standards of quality of work within a profession. Clearly giving feedback on performance and constructive criticism is a central function of management. Regular formal sessions would avoid the tendency to give feedback only where nurses have done something they should not have or omitted to do something they should have done. A clear structure and adherence to boundaries would also help avoid the sessions becoming either a woolly mutual admiration exercise at one extreme or a secular confession at the other. Potential problem areas might appropriately be anticipated or resolved but equally, positive achievements can be acknowledged and the individual would feel valued and respected as a result. Issues of contract, content and boundaries are considered later in this chapter.

FORMATIVE SUPERVISION: ISSUES OF EDUCATION AND PROFESSIONAL DEVELOPMENT

However necessary and valuable such a normative approach might be, a line manager, possibly from a different professional background, may well not be able to help the nurse develop skills, understanding and competence – the formative aspect of clinical supervision. This essentially educational focus would require a supervisor who is certainly an experienced practitioner and preferably experienced in the specific area of practice of the supervisee. Butterworth and

Faugier (1992) underline the need for supervisors to be practitioners rather than managers as such. Catmur (1995) agrees that clinical supervision has more credibility if carried out by someone in contact with the clinical environment on a regular basis.

With this type of clinical supervision, there are significant differences from the normative aspect. First, the supervisor does not have to be the manager. The choice of supervisor could, and indeed some argue it should, remain with the nurse (Devine 1995). Second, the work need not necessarily be undertaken on an individual basis and the supervisor might work with small groups or teams. Two other ways of organizing such supervision might be used: one-to-one peer supervision, where pairs of nurses of similar grades and expertise work together, and network supervision, where a group of people with similar expertise and interests who do not necessarily work in the same area on a day-to-day basis come together to discuss relevant issues (Houston 1990). These approaches would obviously not be appropriate for novice nurses. In one area, however, it was felt that group supervision would be the most appropriate approach to supervision for nurses working with the severely mentally ill (Everitt *et al.* 1996). There was an awareness of the risk of members focusing on negative factors or alternatively avoiding criticism by excessive mutual praise and so small groups were put together with different levels of expertise, each having two facilitators, and a specific contract was established. Such contracts are arguably essential for any type of clinical supervision.

A further significant difference between normative and formative supervision is that with the latter there are a variety of ways in which the work might be structured. Work could centre on casework presentation, which may involve observation of live sessions or sessions recorded on video or audiotape. Alternatively, role play might be used, as well as the more traditional verbal presentation by the nurse, followed by discussion with the supervisor or group. The way in which material is presented must vary, depending on the situation. For example, live observation or role play may be appropriate for looking at skills in rapport building or interviewing but would probably not be for considering the nature of the relationship between the nurse and the client, risk assessment or the management of difficult behaviours such as wandering or incontinence in the elderly, for example. In such cases a 'snapshot' of behaviour and skills would simply not be adequate to identify and explore the range of issues involved.

Formative work may therefore take many forms and use many strategies from simple discussion to action techniques such as role play. However, separating some clinical issues from personal ones may not always prove straightforward.

RESTORATIVE SUPERVISION: ISSUES OF SUPPORT

Mental health nursing rightly places great emphasis on the fact that the main therapeutic tool is the self and the relationship developed with the client. Technology is of no value without humanity. The dividing line between our clinical skills and our personal feelings is therefore a narrow one. Clients may be adorable to some but infuriating to others; the difference must be the experience, perception and attitudes of the individual nurse. For example, some may find it difficult if not impossible to work with clients who abuse children sexually, while others may see such perpetrators as victims themselves, and be well able to work with them effectively. Personal feelings may therefore be very relevant to clinical work in mental health.

Being close to people in distress can itself be distressing. Faugier (1994) compares clinical supervision with 'pit-head time' – the opportunity coal miners have to clean themselves, within work time, before clocking off and going home. She suggests that clinical supervision is the equivalent for those who work 'at the coal face of emotional distress, disease, death, loss and confusion' and that none has a stronger claim for such support than the mental health nurse.

There is also a legal issue relating to support, in that managers have a duty to provide a healthy environment for their workforce. In 1994, in the case of John Edward Walker vs Northumberland County Council, the High Court ruled that the employer was liable for an employee's breakdown as a result of excessive workload. On a more pragmatic level, unless the nurse looks after herself, she is no position to look after others. If in an aeroplane there is a drop in cabin pressure and oxygen masks are needed, parents with small children are told to go against their protective instincts and put their own mask on first; that way they will be able to reassure and if necessary hold the mask on the potentially struggling child. Professionally, if nurses do not acknowledge their own emotional pressures and distress, they are at risk of burning out and being of no further use to their clients. Providing support is a responsibility of the manager, but seeking it is equally a responsibility of the nurse.

The nature of the restorative element of supervision is therefore again important, but with significant differences from the normative and formative aspects. Where normative work is an essential function of management and formative an essential part of professional development, restorative cannot be in any way imposed. The nurse will simply not risk sharing personal material unless she feels comfortable and safe. The links between the elements may, however, be inextricable; if issues of stress in the nurse are not addressed, then the quality of care will be adversely affected (Sullivan 1993).

The restorative element of clinical supervision must therefore be available and facilitated but cannot be imposed, and this can lead to problems. While, for example, the line manager may be clinically credible and therefore able to work with both managerial and clinical issues, nurses would understandably be reluctant to share anxieties about personal issues or those that they feel might adversely affect their career development – from just feeling unmotivated or finding work overwhelming to agonizing about whether to change jobs.

ORGANIZING SUPERVISION

Personal and local needs and situations will naturally vary but there are certain elements that must be considered and each will now be addressed.

- Choice of supervisor
- Ground rules
- Theoretical orientation
- Boundaries
- Structure of sessions
- Documentation
- Confidentiality
- Supervision for the supervisor
- Evaluation mechanism (Everitt *et al.* 1996, Oxley 1995)

Choice of supervisor

Depending on the circumstances, it may not be possible for the nurse to choose her supervisor. If the normative issues are seen as central, then a line manager would be expected to undertake the clinical supervision. Problems might then arise if the nurse talks about practices below the required standard and there is potentially an ethical dilemma relating to confidentiality (Jones 1997). It has been suggested that this role conflict might be alleviated if managers work in partnership with other trusts or the private sector, which could prove beneficial to nurses, managers and clients alike (Lyle 1998), but clearly a high degree of trust would be required in what is still to an extent a competitive market place.

If the nurse is able to choose her supervisor, there are certain factors she might consider. It has been suggested that the supervisor should have skills in communication, be able to be supportive and possess both general and specialist clinical skills (Wilkin, in Butterworth and Faugier 1992). Communication skills would include active listening and giving constructive feedback; supportive skills would involve knowing how and when to give support; general skills would include knowledge about current issues in mental health nursing; and specialist skills are those related to the clinical area or therapeutic activity of the nurse, for example assertive outreach or cognitive-behavioural therapy. Fowler (1996) emphasizes the need for the supervisor to be able to employ a range of interventions, including counselling and educational skills. Some have chosen to emphasize the need for the supervisor to have advanced clinical skills, with the nurse having the opportunity to observe them in practice, as well as being guided in terms of their own interventions (Sloan 1998). Others have felt that the supervisors should be trained in supervision and meet with other supervisors (Jones and Bennett 1998, Wilkin, in Butterworth and Faugier 1992).

The key themes to emerge – the things to look for in a potential supervisor – are that the supervisor should be a competent clinician who is capable of giving specific ideas about interventions in a range of ways within a supportive relationship. In short, the supervisor should be 'supportive, motivational, educative and modelling' (Catmur 1995).

Ground rules

It is crucial that the nature of any clinical supervision arrangement is clearly stated in the form of a contract (Wilkin *et al.* 1997). The administrative aspects must include membership, frequency, duration, location, agenda, content and contingencies. It must be clear exactly who is involved, naturally if any work is undertaken in a group setting. Commitment to attendance is also vital. How often meetings occur and how long they last should be agreed in advance, since *ad hoc* arrangements have a tendency to stop happening, and a location or series of locations should similarly be planned ahead. Agenda and content, for example presenting casework or dealing with urgent matters, should be agreed in principle in advance. The 'what shall we do today?' approach would not endear itself to the busy professional. If supervision is being undertaken on an individual basis, it is still important to agree the process and procedure in advance. Planning for contingencies – what to do if there are unresolved issues, for example – should also be anticipated and agreed between the respective parties.

Theoretical orientation

It is important to be clear about the style of supervision being used. This will also have a bearing on the material being explored and is related to the choice of supervisor. For example, it would be unhelpful for a supervisor to adopt a psychoanalytical approach when considering the work being undertaken in reducing urinary incontinence in an assessment unit for the over-65s. On the other hand, using the principles of client-centred counselling when exploring relationships in the context of counselling may well be helpful.

Boundaries

As with other aspects, the specific boundaries will vary, depending on the chosen focus. If normative or managerial, then the agenda will probably be established by the supervisor, with specific areas to be addressed – for example, maintenance of standards of care. If the main focus is formative or educational, then it might be appropriate to limit work to issues relating to client care only, with general administrative issues at one end and personal issues at the other being excluded. It is not always easy to divorce professional from personal issues with clients; it has been suggested that personal material should be brought into the session if it affects or is affected by the work being discussed (Hawkins and Shohet 1989). If the work is primarily restorative or supportive, then arguably the focus should be on personal or emotional rather than administrative or clinical issues, although McCallion and Baxter (1995) found that one concern about clinical supervision among nurses was that it might be a form of compulsory therapy, stirring up powerful feelings against their wishes. A study of the topics addressed in supervision across a range of sites found there to be a wide range, including organizational issues, clinical skills, career advice, educational support, confidence building, interpersonal problems and personal matters (Butterworth *et al.* 1997). The question of whether it is possible to blend satisfactorily all three elements of clinical supervision within one contact is a difficult one.

Structure of session

The structure could include both an agenda and agreed time limit but must have a degree of flexibility. It would be absurd to prevent a nurse from talking about a suicide that had happened the day before simply because the previous week it had been agreed that a different problem would be presented.

Within each session there are any number of headings that might be used – a case presentation or critical incident analysis, for example. There is a range of models to choose from. For example, Boud's five stages of reflection (Boud 1985) consider the trigger (the reason the subject was chosen); the description (the detail of context and behaviour); the analysis (the discussion of feelings and acknowledge); developing new perspectives; and deciding on a plan of action. This is not dissimilar from Egan's counselling model (1990), where clients are helped to explore the present scenario, develop a preferred scenario and plan how to achieve their aims. It is perhaps best to choose a model that links with the nature of the work being undertaken in the clinical area.

Documentation

There must be no doubt about who is keeping records of what. It may be that for individual work the nurse keeps a reflective diary or clinical journal (Brown and Sorrell 1993) or for group work the supervisor records information such as attendance and any conclusions reached (Everitt *et al.* 1996). It has also been suggested that it may be beneficial if the supervisor makes notes in the early stages of the work (Butcher 1995) or indeed that record keeping is important in demonstrating commitment and helping the reflective process (Devine 1995). It is also important to establish how any documentation may be used; for example, in evaluating the nurse's development or reviewing the supervisory process.

Confidentiality

Classically, information is not released outside the session other than on a need-to-know basis. As discussed above, there may be problems with role conflict if issues are raised relating to problems with quality or standards of practice. It is important that rules of confidentiality are made clear at the outset, to minimize difficulties establishing trust within the supervisory relationship. It should be made explicit that matters relating to pay, promotion or discipline should not be included in the supervisory process (Kohner 1994).

Supervision for the supervisor

Supervision should be available for all practitioners at all levels (UKCC 1996). In order to maintain standards and to support the supervisors, they should receive both training and supervision for that aspect of their work. The nature of this supervision should be clarified, as it will have a bearing on issues of confidentiality and trust.

Evaluation mechanisms

A time and mechanism should be agreed for an evaluation of the supervisory relationship. The evaluation or review, however, may highlight issues which lead to changes in the supervision contract. Individual sessions as well as a series of sessions may be reviewed. There should, however, be no insistence on the part of anyone involved that the work continue to the point of evaluation, come what may.

Problems with implementation

Clinical supervision, of whatever focus, involves an investment – investing work time in staff, rather than patient contact, whether to monitor performance, develop skills or provide emotional support – and this investment is the time of the supervisor as well as the nurse. There is much anecdotal evidence of the effectiveness of supervision (Everitt *et al.* 1996) and some specific research has suggested that there is sufficient evidence to show that clinical supervision has an impact on practitioners and the way they work (Butterworth *et al.* 1997).

In addition to the organization finding the funding, the individuals finding the time and suitably skilled supervisors being available, there is a range of potential problems in getting the work off the ground. Mention has already been made of the anxieties of nurses – that supervision will either furnish their management with evidence against them or they will be forced to explore feelings or personal issues they would prefer not to. Another possibility is the risk of feeling deskilled; the idea that as weaknesses are pointed out they will be made to feel useless. This is related to a denial of the need to change practice, similar to the individuals avoiding going to the dentist, in case some work actually needs doing. Ignorance is not always bliss. On another level, many studies have argued that implementing clinical supervision is intuitively a sound and productive exercise but these have been more anecdotal than empirical (Rogers 1998).

It may be difficult to argue for the development of clinical supervision without hard evidence for its effectiveness and a clear definition of focus and approach. It could mean a mini-appraisal interview, studies of casework in groups or an exploration of psychodynamic aspects of therapeutic relationships. Many have said 'it' is a good idea but there are also many interpretations of what 'it' actually is. It is perhaps more helpful to return to the three main aspects and acknowledge that each might best be explored in a different way.

The normative aspect could therefore be undertaken by meetings on a regular basis with the line manager, planned rather than *ad hoc*, where it is possible to acknowledge and build on strengths while standards are monitored and any specific personal goals agreed. Such goals should be SMART – Specific, Measurable, Attainable, Relevant and Trackable (Blanchard 1987) – which is consistent with any goals negotiated with clients.

The formative element of supervision demands a supervisor who is credible in clinical practice and flexible in terms of the strategies used to help the nurse develop skills and explore specific clinical difficulties. Ideally the nurse will choose such a supervisor who, in addition to clinical and educational expertise, will have similar skills to those used by a counsellor (Devine 1995) – someone who can 'listen, counsel, and guide' (Eddison 1994).

The restorative element of supervision is the one which must be available in some form but, perhaps paradoxically, cannot be imposed and nurses should be able to choose their supervisor. Rogers (1998), while acknowledging evidence that clinical supervision might reduce staff stress, suggests that if the aim is indeed to reduce stress, then 'We should help staff develop stress management skills' which would be less costly than dealing with the issue through clinical supervision. There are many well-established stress management skills, including time management, assertiveness, relaxation, breathing training, diet and exercise, positive thinking, and giving and receiving support (Gournay 1995, Makin 1991). Indeed, there are well over 100 other strategies or therapies for managing stress, some more empirically proven than others (Alexander 1996). Many of the established strategies will require the individual nurse to address issues in the workplace, so the notion that teaching sessions on strategies and enabling the nurse to get on with things can occur without this impacting on the work environment is optimistic, bordering on the naive.

It is essential that the humanity central to mental health nursing is not ignored. The stress is intrinsically related to clinical work; working with clients' thoughts, feelings and behaviours is demanding and exhausting (Simms 1992). It is surely a positive and helpful move to provide support for the nurse in the form of a relationship where unresolved feelings arising as a consequence of caring are 'exposed, examined and dissipated' (Sloan 1998). It is arguable that if nurses feel cared for, they will in turn feel more positive in their caring for others.

While the restorative issues are therefore important, there is a range of ways in which such support may be implemented. Given that mental health nurses should all have at least a grounding in the principles and practice of counselling, it is feasible to use peers or colleagues as a resource in this area. This process therefore offers the opportunity both to talk through personal issues and to develop skills in facilitation. Cynics might argue that this could degenerate into idle gossip or a situation where 'the blind lead the blind' but if properly structured, such a process could prove to be a sound investment. John Heron describes such a process as 'co-counselling'. He regards it as an opportunity to explore and learn from experience and to develop counselling skills in a safe environment. It is a two-way process among peers, each taking a turn as facilitator (or supervisor) and client. The client is the nurse at the centre of the process, exploring her experiences and celebrating skills, with the facilitator giving support, through active listening and empathic response. Empathy is central to the process (see Chapter 4) while neither apathy nor sympathy is helpful.

As with any approach to work in supervision, it is important to establish a contract specifying issues as discussed above, including ground rules, boundaries, structure, documentation, confidentiality and evaluation. The work should be undertaken in work time. It is important to have personal as well as organizational commitment; if one nurse devotes time but the other fails to do so, the first will feel devalued, if not rejected.

It may be helpful for such work to be supervised by a more experienced supervisor from time to time, certainly in the early stages. Some guidelines for both roles in the process might be given, the most important aspect being the timing of the session, specifically for how long each person adopts the supervisory role. Other guidelines for the facilitator might include suggesting that they **do**:

- ask for clarification
- reflect feelings
- paraphrase
- use silence
- give full attention
- use non-verbal active listening techniques
- demonstrate understanding
- encourage positive perceptions

but endeavour **not to**:

- interpret
- advise
- criticize or blame
- instruct
- chat
- deny feelings
- plan what to say while the other is talking.

Equivalent, in the position of client, the nurse might be encouraged to **try to**:

- celebrate good experiences
- acknowledge personal qualities
- express feelings and use 'I' when you mean 'I' (rather than 'you', 'we' or 'one')
- think creatively
- be specific

and advised **not to**:

- underestimate skills or qualities or be inappropriately modest
- dismiss feelings
- dismiss compliments
- apologize excessively
- give up if details cannot be remembered or anxiety is experienced.

Whilst it is difficult to qualify what constitutes 'good' support for nurses at work, it has been suggested that qualities often associated with humanistic counselling must be relevant – warmth, concern for feelings and not being defensive or impatient, for example. Specifically, if the nurse feels respected and understood in terms of empathy, this seems to be a factor in reducing stress and emotional exhaustion (Firth *et al.* 1986). This process is not barefoot therapy; however, the notion that we can learn about caring from the way in which we are cared for is important. If the organization provides time and space for the process and nurses value and in turn feel valued by that organization, this will surely have positive repercussions in terms of valuing their clients, consistent with the need for those who supervise to themselves be supervised.

This is not the same, however, as the notion that unless you have personally experienced something, you will not be able effectively to work with someone in that situation. The experience of being cared for is positive and this can be extended to caring for others. Although this is a transferable or generalizable skill, this does not mean that it is impossible to work with someone with whom the nurse does not have common experience. It is clearly possible to work, for example, with someone who is depressed without having been depressed oneself. Most important, perhaps, is the ability to be sensitive in the work with that person, noting similarities and acknowledging differences. It is essential to avoid jumping to conclusions, without knowing how other people feel. It is dangerous at least, and disastrous at worst, to try to short-circuit the development of a relationship by naively, albeit with all good intentions, simply saying 'I know how you feel'. This is a principle which applies whether discussing issues with colleagues or with clients.

CONCLUSION

While much has been written about the benefits of clinical supervision, there are problems implementing it in such a way that all its aims are achieved. In mental health nursing, with its focus on the nurse–client relationship, there are particularly good reasons for offering all nurses all aspects of clinical supervision. Working with vulnerable clients demands systems to ensure safety and quality of care. Equally, working with people in distress is itself distressing and support must be available if cynicism or emotional burnout is to be avoided. Effective supervision demands an investment at individual and organizational level. There is no doubt that such an investment can be of enormous benefit.

REFERENCES

Alexander, J. (1996) *Supertherapies*. Bantam Books, London.

Barber, P. and Norman, I. (1987) An eclectic model of staff development supervision techniques to prepare nurses for a process approach: a social perspective. In: Barber, P. (ed.) *Mental Handicap*. Hodder & Stoughton, Sevenoaks.

Bishop, V. (1994) Clinical supervision for an accountable profession. *Nursing Times* 90(39): 35–39.

Blanchard, K. (1987) *Leadership and the One Minute Manager*. Fontana, London.

Boud, D. (1985) *Reflection: turning experience into learning*. Kogan Page, London.

Brown, H.N. and Sorrell, J. (1993) Use of clinical journals to enhance critical thinking. *Nurse Educator* 18(5): 16–19.

Butcher, K. (1995) Taking notes. *Nursing Times* 91(26): 33.

Butterworth, C.A. and Faugier, J. (1992) *Clinical Supervision and Mentorship in Nursing*. Chapman and Hall, London.

Butterworth, C.A., Carson, J. and White, E. (1997) *It is Good to Talk*. School of Nursing, Midwifery and Health Visiting, University of Manchester.

Casement, P. (1985) *On Learning from the Patient.* Tavistock, London.

Catmur, S. (1995) Clinical supervision in mental health nursing. *Mental Health Nursing* 15(1): 24–25.

DoH (1994) *The Allitt Inquiry: Report of the Independent Inquiry Relating to the Deaths and Inquiries on the Children's Ward at Grantham and Kesteven General Hospital During the Period February to April 1991.* HMSO, London.

Devine, A. (1995) Introducing clinical supervision: a guide. *Nursing Standard* 9(40): 32–34.

Driscoll, J. (1996) Reflection and the management of community nursing practice. *British Journal of Community Health Nursing* 1: 2.

Eddison, G. (1994) Monitoring, mentoring. *Nursing Standard* 8(30): 99.

Egan, G. (1990) *The Skills Helper,* 4th edn. Brooks Cole, Monterey.

Everitt, J., Bradshaw, T. and Butterworth, C.A. (1996) Stress and clinical supervision in mental health care. *Nursing Times* 92(10): 34–35.

Faugier, J. (1994) Thin on the ground. *Nursing Times* 90(20): 64–65.

Firth, W.B., McIntee, I., McKeown, P. and Britton, P. (1986) Interpersonal support amongst nurses at work. *Journal of Advanced Nursing* 11: 273–282.

Fowler, J. (1996) Clinical supervision: what do you say after saying hello? *British Journal of Nursing* 5(6): 382–385.

Gournay, K. (1995) *Stress Management: a guide to coping with stress.* Asset Books, Dorking.

Hawkins, P. and Shohet, R. (1989) *Supervision in the Helping Professions.* Open University Press, Milton Keynes.

Houston, G. (1990) *Supervision and Counselling.* Rochester Foundation, London.

Jones, A. (1997) Communication at the heart of supervision. *Nursing Times* 93(49): 50–51.

Jones, M. and Bennett, J. (1998) Clinical supervision: mental health nurses' views. *Mental Health Practice* 2(4): 18–22.

Kohner, H. (1994) *Clinical Supervision in Practice.* King's Fund Centre, London.

Luft, J. (1984) *Group Process: an introduction to group dynamics* 3rd edn. National Press Book, Palo Alto.

Lyle, D. (1998) Can nursing managers supervise?. *Nursing Times* 2(7): 8.

Makin, P. (1991) *Positive Stress Management.* Kogan Page, London.

Marken, M. and Payne, M. (eds) (1986) *Enabling and Ensuring.* National Youth Bureau and Council for Education and Training in Youth and Community Work, Leicester.

McCallion, H. and Baxter, T. (1995) Clinical supervision – how it works in the real world. *Nursing Management* 1(9): 20–21.

NHS Management Executive (1993) *A Vision for the Future.* Department of Health, London.

Oxley, P. (1995) Clinical supervision in community psychiatric nursing. *Mental Health Nursing* 13(6): 15–17.

Rogers, P. (1998) Hype that is hard to swallow. *Mental Health Practice* 1(10): 18.

Scanlon, C. and Weir, W.S. (1997) Learning from practice? Mental health nurses' perceptions and experiences of clinical supervision. *Journal of Advanced Nursing* 26: 295–303.

Simms, J. (1992) Supervision. In: Wright, H. and Giddy, M. (eds) *Mental Health Nursing.* Chapman and Hall, London.

Sloan, G. (1998) Clinical supervision: characteristics of a good supervisor. *Nursing Standard* 12(40): 42–46.

Sullivan, P. (1993) Occupational stress in psychiatric nursing. *Journal of Advanced Nursing* 18: 591–601.

UKCC (1996) *Position Statement on Clinical Supervision for Nursing and Health Visiting.* UKCC, London.

Wilkin, P., Bowers, L. and Monk, J. (1997) Clinical supervision: managing the resistance. *Nursing Times* 93(8): 48–49.

8 THE NURSE AS RESEARCHER

Doug MacInnes

OBJECTIVES

After reading this chapter, you should be able to:

- identify that research is one of a number of methods by which mental health nurses develop knowledge
- list the different components of the research process
- understand the principles for critically appraising research studies and apply this appraisal to clinical practice
- identify the information needed when writing a research proposal
- list areas that need to be considered when writing up a research study
- identify potential areas for research.

INTRODUCTION

This chapter examines the value and the process of undertaking research within mental health nursing. Its main concern is to give a brief understanding of the ways in which research design can be appraised as well as giving some indication of research projects that are currently being developed within mental health nursing. The chapter is not intended to be a complete guide giving information about every aspect of research. Instead, it concentrates on the basics of the research process and some of the most important components of this process. This includes a description of the components that need to be incorporated when detailing a research proposal and those that need to be considered when writing a research report. It will also give a brief overview of the development of research within mental health nursing and also discuss some of the possible areas for future research.

Research in nursing is part of the role of every nurse. The UKCC *Code of Conduct* (1996) states that it is the responsibility of every nurse to ensure that the care given is fully informed. This means that it is the professional duty of all nurses to ensure that they are up to date with the current research in their area of practice. However, research is only one way in which mental health nurses gain knowledge and before looking specifically at research, Robson (1997) noted that nurses also gain knowledge through the following:

- ritual
- trial and error

- experience
- intuition.

Ritual

This can be defined as any action that involves more or less mechanical or unvarying performance of certain activities. It is seen to be caused by frequent repetition of tasks which may lead to action without thought. The ritual of the medication ward round can be seen as one instance within mental health nursing. The rationale for maintaining ward rounds at set times is unclear in the majority of ward areas and yet the practice continues in most cases.

Trial and error and experience

This involves the development of ways of working through either experiencing successful outcomes with particular interventions or trying different ways of working until one way seems to bring about a positive conclusion. The same actions are then repeated for each new case. An example might be that it is found that an aroused client can be calmed by the staff using distracting techniques to stop the client focusing on particular thoughts or feelings. This technique may then be used on other clients when the need arises to deescalate situations. If the approach is successful in the majority of situations, the nursing staff may decide to use it when any client becomes aroused.

Knowledge is developed in this way because it is relatively easy to learn this approach as it is part of the everyday culture and practice of the nursing environment and is seen, if part of a ward/team philosophy, as a socially acceptable way of learning and practising. Some limitations of this method are that the application of the knowledge and the rationale behind it are localized. This approach can be haphazard and unsystematic in nature, making it hard to distinguish which part of the approach is successful. It also presupposes that individual practitioners are experienced enough to be able to identify the positive and negative aspects of any potential outcomes. There is also the danger of nursing practice becoming static and ritualistic care becoming established.

Intuition

On occasions nursing knowledge and behaviour are not based on logical or rational thought and consequently the reason for actions cannot be explained. This intuitive knowledge arises because expertise in given situations or encounters leads to internalization of why and how actions occur. An example might be a nurse confronted with a client who is shouting and threatening to cause physical harm to the nurse. If the nurse is experienced in dealing with violent incidents she may be able to intuitively assess the potential danger of the situation without needing to consciously consider the various individual elements.

The only concern with this knowledge-based approach is that an overreliance on intuitive knowledge and an underreliance on a rational decision-making process means that the individual components of the knowledge underpinning individual practice are not obvious, leading to the expertise remaining within individual nurses.

Research

Research is the most formalized way of gaining knowledge and is often used in conjunction with the other ways of obtaining knowledge noted above. In many cases, mental health nurses' experiences, behaviours and intuitions will lead on to research activities and will also influence their perceptions as to the validity of published research articles. Nursing research has been defined as an attempt to increase the sum of what is known, usually referred to as a body of knowledge, by the discovery of new facts or relationships through a process of systematic enquiry – the research process (MacLeod-Clark and Hockey 1989). This is a formal process with individual stages that gives a clear and precise method for establishing the reliability and validity of new and existing practices within mental health nursing.

However, we should remember that intuition and experience can guide nurses as to the sense research can make. If mental health nursing research is not perceived as intuitively correct or it does not correspond to a nurse's experiences, the nurse may not see the research conclusions as either valid or useful.

REASONS FOR NURSING RESEARCH

The purpose of research in nursing has been described by Cormack (1996) as increasing the sum of what is known about the professional activity of nurses, which may be in nursing education, nursing administration or nursing practice in its many forms and settings. This is undoubtedly true though the definition does not include the fact that nurses, and mental health nurses in particular, develop areas of research into new areas of practice and interest. The Thorn Initiative is a case in point (Brooker *et al.* 1994). This was developed by nurses and other disciplines to address the lack of skills that had been found in CPNs when dealing with the seriously mentally ill. This had been documented by the quinquennial CPN survey of 1990 (White 1990). A training programme focusing on developing skills in family work, cognitive-behavioural work and case management was devised and research undertaken by the organizers of the training to ascertain the efficacy of this programme. The results showed that this new type of intervention with clients and their families was effective in reducing admission rates and enhancing the client's quality of life (Brooker et al. 1994).

It is within this framework that nursing research can enhance the knowledge, skills and options of practitioners and academic nurses in their endeavour to ensure the highest quality of care for patients and their families.

The main purposes of nursing research are listed by Cormack (1969) as follows.

- To establish scientifically defensible reasons for nursing activities.
- To provide nurses with an increased repertoire of scientifically defensible nursing intervention options.

- To find ways of increasing the cost effectiveness of nursing activities.
- To provide a basis for standard setting and quality assurance.
- To provide evidence in support of demands for resources in nursing.
- To satisfy the academic curiosity of thinking nurses.
- To facilitate interdisciplinary collaboration in health-care research.
- To facilitate multinational collaboration in nursing and nursing research.
- To earn and defend a professional status for nursing.

HISTORICAL DEVELOPMENT OF NURSING RESEARCH

Research has been a part of the way that nurses organize and evaluate their practice since Florence Nightingale carried out her epidemiological research into infection control within the military camps in the Crimea and established an association with the number of fatalities.

However, in the 100 years between 1850 and 1950 the nursing index on research comprised only two volumes and the studies it contained consisted primarily of descriptions of the roles that nurses undertook in the course of their work. In the 1950s the number of nursing studies increased (mainly in the USA) though these were still mainly descriptive with a limited theoretical base. From the 1970s onwards a greater concentration of nursing studies has been reported with many focusing on the effectiveness of nursing care and examination of clients' needs. These developments have been clearly related to both government and public concerns relating to the cost effectiveness of health care.

The development of nursing research in Britain was also enhanced by the increasing amount of research and critical analysis that was included in nurse training curricula. However, it was not until 1956 that the first nurse in Britain obtained a PhD and not until 1960 that the first nurse training PhD course was established in Edinburgh. Until recently most nursing PhDs have been obtained through medical schools. The change of nurse training base from hospital school of nursing to higher education also helped in the development of research appreciation and research skills. These developments have both increased the research awareness of nurses and also helped to introduce into the nursing arena clinical practices based on findings from research undertaken by nurses.

Mental health nursing research

The NHSE (1997) defined that the future of the health service lay in creating a knowledge-based service in which clinical, managerial and policy decisions were based on sound information about research findings and scientific developments. To achieve this within the mental health field, nurses have to show through reading, appraising and undertaking research that their actions and interventions are effective and can be clearly evaluated as such. Although the evidence is limited, studies into the readiness of mental health nurses to function in this role show that there are still limitations in the research skills and experience is needed.

A survey of Parahoo (1999) (Table 8.1) showed that in comparison to general nurses, mental health nurses were less likely to utilize research. This is supported by the results from Table 8.2 that show that even though mental health nurses state that they are more knowledgeable about the principles of undertaking a research study, they are less likely to implement research findings in clinical practice.

If both tables are taken into consideration, it can be seen that, although they are aware of the basic principles of research, the majority of mental health nurses are unable to critique a research report or evaluate how research could be use in practice.

In terms of the types of research that mental health nurses undertake, Yonge *et al.* (1996) examined all the literature within a range of psychiatric journals over a 10-year period with the eligibility criteria being that at least one of the authors was a mental health nurse. The findings show only a few mental health nurses publishing research articles with only 194 articles meeting the criteria set by the authors out of a total of 3900 articles reviewed. It is interesting to note that nearly half of the research found was quantitative (94 in total) in nature. This is in contrast to Cullum's (1998) findings that overall over 75% of all research in nursing is qualitative. This gives the overall view that mental health

Table 8.1 Research utilization by nurses (Parahoo 1999)

Frequency	RGN (%)	RMN (%)
Never	2.8	8.8
Seldom	5	9.5
Sometimes	53.1	53.7
Frequency	29.1	20.1
All the time	6.9	4.4
No response	3	3.4

Table 8.2 Extent of research preparation (Parahoo 1999)

Activity	RGN (%)	RMN (%)
Appreciate the contributions of research to practice	54.7	52.4
Understand the basic principles of research	51.6	58.7
Write a research proposal	26.8	30.3
Carry out a small-scale project	26.5	35.3
Use libraries to access research–based material	57.5	63.1
Evaluate/critique research articles/reports	35.7	40.8
Use research-based information in practice	53.7	41.7
Implement research findings in practice	48	38.8

nurses are less likely to publish research than general nurses, but are proportionally more likely to publish quantitative research.

For an examination of the potential reasons behind the lack of published research from mental health nurses, an analysis of a recent report *Addressing Acute Concerns* may be of benefit. The report was published in 1999 by the Standing Nursing and Midwifery Advisory Committee (SNMAC) and reported to the government about the developing role of the mental health nurse and the contribution of nurses to the provision of modern mental health acute care. The report contained 44 references with only 15 of these being references where at least one was a nurse. There were only six nursing articles where specific research reports were noted as opposed to 14 research reports referenced from other disciplines. The majority of the nursing research reports referenced were done in conjunction with other disciplines (mainly psychiatrists and/or psychologists). In addition, most of the nursing research reported came from one higher education institution. This indicates that the published research is limited in both quantity and that it is concentrated within specific institutions.

A further concern can be noted when examining how nursing research is reported. The programme of a major nursing conference, the 10th biennial conference of the Workgroup of European Nurse Researchers (WENR 2000), contained over 150 research papers from nurses from across Europe and North America. However, only eight focused on mental health issues. This gives further indications that mental health nurses are less likely than other nursing groups to both document and present any research that is undertaken. There seems to be a reluctance and/or a lack of opportunity to undertake research without assistance from other professional disciplines, most notably psychiatry and psychology. There is also a dearth of joint research between mental health nurses and other nursing specialities even though certain areas may prove fruitful for this type of joint study. Major large-scale research studies and studies requiring substantial resources are more likely to be undertaken by nurses within a multidisciplinary approach. This is because these types of research studies require high numbers of participants and also large amounts of financial and other resources to support the study. This can only realistically be done through different disciplines combining their talents and experiences or by the research being supervised by a health researcher with a proven good research record.

The document *Achieving Effective Practice* which was published by the NHSE (1999a) establishes a criteria by which nurses can measure effective clinical practice in the workplace. It put forward the view that knowledge about research was of central importance in developing effective and valid change within nursing practice. The main skills that nurses needed were the abilities to develop a research proposal and to write a research report. The acquisition of knowledge and skills in these two areas allowed nurse researchers to obtain support for their research project and develop a clearly focused research design and enabled the findings to be widely disseminated and clearly understood. The more research nurses were able to undertake, the more experience and expertise they were likely to acquire and the greater the opportunity to develop contacts to advance further research.

This chapter examines the processes involved in developing a research proposal and writing a research report. However, before describing this, it is beneficial to distinguish the various components of the research process as these guide the structure and content of both research proposals and reports.

THE RESEARCH PROCESS

Most definitions of research state that its main emphasis is the obtaining of new knowledge through a predetermined systematic process – the research process. Although Parahoo's (1999) study suggests that over half of qualified mental health nurses are aware of the research process it is perhaps prudent to restate its main principles. The stages of the research process are briefly noted below and follow the order in which they are generally recorded within a research report.

- Title
- Author(s)
- Abstract
- Introduction
- Literature review
- Hypothesis
- Operational definitions
- Methodology
- Subjects
- Sample selection
- Data collection
- Ethical considerations
- Results
- Data analysis
- Discussion
- Conclusions
- Recommendations

The strengths and weaknesses of each area need to be recognized before a piece of research can be critically appraised. It is not within the scope of this chapter to discuss in detail all the areas mentioned above but some of the more important stages will be deliberated.

LITERATURE REVIEW

A review of the literature is an objective criticism based upon factual material and supported by appropriate evidence and argument. It notes the positive and negative aspects of the material. The implications of any flaws identified in previous works are also highlighted. It should create a structure upon which further research can be based and then used when discussing research findings.

Where to find the literature

The literature relevant to the research to be undertaken can be found in many areas. The increasing importance of the World Wide Web has led to developments being reported in increasing numbers and reports are available online soon after the research has been completed. However, the research report may not be subject to the same scientific scrutiny as a paper published in either a reputable journal or a book. The list below gives some ideas of where to find relevant literature.

- Journals
- Books
- Reports
- Theses
- Conference proceedings
- Government documents
- Computer databases (CD-ROMs)
- Internet
- Library
- Fellow health professionals

The ability to conduct a literature review is important both to find out what other research has been done (or not done) in a specific clinical area and also to find information on measures and research procedures used in previous research which can help nurses when developing future research projects.

The procedure for undertaking a literature review is shown in Figure 8.1.

Once a literature review has been undertaken, nurses can examine certain criteria to assess the validity of their literature review.

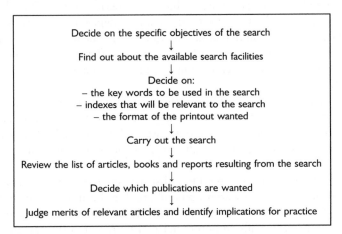

Decide on the specific objectives of the search
↓
Find out about the available search facilities
↓
Decide on:
– the key words to be used in the search
– indexes that will be relevant to the search
– the format of the printout wanted
↓
Carry out the search
↓
Review the list of articles, books and reports resulting from the search
↓
Decide which publications are wanted
↓
Judge merits of relevant articles and identify implications for practice

Figure 8.1   How to conduct a literature search (NHSE 1999a)

- *Current knowledge* – the review should contain up-to-date literature.
- The *underlying theoretical frameworks* need to be clearly stated – an example would be that if a person was undertaking research using a family systems approach, the constructs underpinning family systems theory would need to be explained.
- A *balanced view* – the review should present a critical analysis of the positive and negative aspects of any theory, methodology or approach discussed within the review.
- *Need for research* – the review should identify the reason why the research is justified.

RESEARCH DESIGN

The design is the researcher's overall plan for obtaining answers to research questions and testing the research hypothesis (if a hypothesis has been put forward). A hypothesis is a testable statement that relates to the researcher's expectations of the variables under consideration of the study. If a nurse wanted to examine the effectiveness of a supportive counselling approach to a group of clients with depression, a potential hypothesis might be that using a supportive counselling approach reduces the level of depression. In some types of research, usually qualitative research, a problem statement may be used instead of a hypothesis. This is less specific than a hypothetical statement and usually focuses on giving a broad overview about the phenomena under investigation. A problem statement in the above example might be that the study examined the relationship between supportive counselling and its effect on a group of depressed clients.

The research design should also state the research approach that is to be adopted. There are a number of different approaches that can be used in mental health nursing, which will be documented below. The two main differences are between quantitative and qualitative research. In quantitative research the information obtained is primarily measurable in numerical form. This differs from qualitative research which seeks to gain an in-depth investigation of human phenomena in order to understand the values and meanings these phenomena have for the individuals under study. The main differences between these two paradigms in practice have been documented by Burns and Grove (1993) and are shown in Box 8.1.

The researcher needs to decide whether a quantitative or a qualitative design is more likely to answer the research question. They are two different philosophies but are not necessarily polar opposites. Elements of both designs can be used together in mixed-methods studies to provide more information than could be obtained by using either one alone.

Another contrast that is sometimes distinguished is the difference between two types of quantitative research (experimental and non-experimental). Experimental research is where the researcher actively institutes an intervention as part of the research project while in non-experimental research the researcher gathers data without trying to bring about any changes.

Box 8.1 **Differences between quantitative and qualitative methodology (Burns and Grove 1993)**

Quantitative	Qualitative
Objective	Subjective
'Hard' science	'Soft' science
Literature review must be done early in study	Literature review may be done as study progresses or afterwards
Tests theory	Develops theory
One reality: focus is concise and narrow	Multiple realities: focus is complex and broad
Reduction, control, precision	Discovery, description, understanding, shared interpretation
Measurable	Interpretative
Mechanistic: parts equal the whole	Organismic: whole is greater than the parts
Report: statistical analysis. Basic element of analysis is numbers	Report rich narrative individual interpretation. Basic element of analysis is words/ideas
Researcher is separate	Researcher is part of process
Subjects	Participants
Context free	Context dependent
Hypothesis	Research questions
Reasoning is logical and deductive	Reasoning is dialectic and inductive
Establishes relationships, causation	Describes meaning, discovery
Uses instruments	Uses communication and observation
Strives for generalization	Strives for uniqueness
Designs: descriptive, correlational quasi-experimental, experimental	Designs: phenomenological, grounded theory, ethnographic, historical philosophical, case study
Sample size: 30 to 500	Sample size is not a concern: seeks 'information-rich' sample
'Counts the beans'	Provides information as to 'which beans are worth counting'

Three examples will now be documented to show the different types of research design described above: experimental, non-experimental and qualitative.

An example of *experimental* research is Carpenter *et al.*'s (1999) study of the efficacy of diazepam treatment when a person with schizophrenia starts to exhibit the first stages of symptom exacerbation. The study population was 53 patients who met the diagnostic criteria of having either schizophrenia or schizoaffective disorder. All the patients were randomly assigned to one of three groups (one having diazepam treatment, one having fluphenazine treatment and one having a placebo effect). The patients' mental states were assessed using the Brief Psychiatric Rating Scale (BPRS) and the Clinical Global Impression (CGI). The patients were assessed before the drug interventions and after a four-week treatment period, using statistical analysis. The results showed that diazepam treatment was statistically superior to placebo treatment and equally as effective as fluohenazine in halting symptom exacerbation. The authors' discussion focused on the usefulness of diazepam in the treatment of prodromal symptoms in schizophrenia as well as when dealing with patients who are reluctant to accept traditional antipsychotic medication.

Within this example, the number of subjects was sufficient for statistical analysis to occur. In addition, the subjects were randomly assigned to either the experimental or intervention group and there was a strict control over the influences that might affect the results of the study. This ensured that the only difference between the three groups was one group having gluphenazine and the other group having a placebo treatment. From this, any differences found could be attributed to the treatments received.

A *non-experimental* case example is described by MacInnes (1998) who examined the views of health services staff as to their perceptions of the levels of burden being faced by relatives and informal caregivers of people with schizophrenia. Forty four health professionals rated their perception of the severity of caregiver burden based on reading 60 direct quotes from caregivers. The severity of the burden was rated on a nine-point rating scale. A score of one equated to the view that the burden experienced would not be stressful while a score of nine would indicate that there would be severe burden. The results obtained showed that in the majority of cases, there were only small differences between different subgroups in relation to the levels of burden that the health professionals apportioned to the caregivers. However, there were a number of differences related to gender, with female professionals rating burdens as significantly more severe when focusing on burdens examining patient behaviours and also annoyance with health services. In addition, nurses were more likely to rate annoyance with health services and burdens relating to patient violence as significantly more severe than did other health professionals. The discussion centred on possible reasons for these differences and also the need for some consistency in the levels of appraisal by different health professionals.

This study had a number of subjects which again allows for statistical analysis to occur. However, the sample were not randomly allocated into two groups, nor was there any intervention. There was less control over other influences that may affect the results. This means that the authors were only able to discuss the possible relationships between variables, but could not make any findings that disclose cause and effect.

A *qualitative* case study example was noted by Lepola and Vanhanen (1997) who studied patients' daily activities within an acute psychiatric ward, by observing the patients in the ward over an extended period of time. Three types of observation were used: general observation, focused observation and selective observation. One of the research team gathered all the data through this approach. The study commenced with 450 hours of general observation which gave a general overview of the ward routine and nursing practice. This was recorded by the researcher through the use of field notes and diaries. Seventy nine hours of focused observation were then undertaken based on the following questions: (a) what type of activities make up the patient's day on an acute psychiatric ward? and (b) how much time do patients spend in the different activities? Finally, seven patients were selected from the initial observations. This was to examine nursing staff's lack of knowledge about patient activities on the ward.

The results were analysed using the constant comparative method. This method is similar to the grounded theory approach in that relationships between concepts and categories are defined, with new information adding to or refining the model or theory. The final results from the study showed that being a patient on an acute psychiatric ward consisted of:

- being alone without any goal-orientated activity
- being alone while participating in the daily routines together with other patients
- acting together with a nurse on the patient's request
- acting together on the nurse's initiative or in the daily routines of the ward.

It can be seen that this research was much more subjective than the two quantitative research designs with the researcher playing an important role in the development of the study. There were fewer subjects, with the emphasis being on nurses' interpretations of the activities subjects, with the emphasis being on nurses' interpretations of the activities being undertaken on the ward and a more in-depth description of these activities. Due to the fact that this study was based on a single ward over an extended period of time, it is less likely that it could be repeated by other nurses nor can its results be generalized to other wards.

Nurses should use research literature to find and evaluate evidence about the effectiveness of nursing interventions and implementing new or different clinical practices. The essential component is nurses' ability to judge whether a research study is relevant to their own area of practice. The NHS (1999a) suggests that there are two approaches to assessing the relevance of studies:

- through individual nurses appraising the literature that they find
- through systematic reviews in which others have critically appraised a range of research studies within a clinical area.

In general terms, nurses are able to gauge whether research is relevant by looking at research studies and judging whether the conclusions reached have some connection to day-to-day practice issues. The judgements are based on what is accepted as good research practice (Polit and Hungler 1993). The NHS

(1999a) state that the three most important questions are:

- Is the research done in the right way?
- Are the research methods and findings of the research relevant to your practice?
- Should you apply what was learned from the research to your clinical practice?

When appraising a research report; three stages are undertaken.

- Was the research design consistent with its purpose?
- Was the research carried out correctly?
- Are the research findings and conclusions consistent?

These three issues are now examined in more detail.

Critical appraisal of research design

There are fairly consistent areas that need to be examined when appraising the design of a research article (Burns and Grove 1993, Hek *et al.* 1996, Parahoo 1997, Polit and Hungler 1993).

1. Does the title tell you what the research is about?
2. Are the reasons/aims of the research clearly stated? *Is the rationale clearly stated? Are the research objectives and/or the hypotheses clearly stated?*
3. Is the review of the literature comprehensive? *Is the literature up to date? Does the literature identify the need for a study? Are you aware of any important references that have been omitted?*
4. Is the sample appropriate? *Is the study population clearly defined? Is there a clear description of how the sample was selected? Are the way the sample was selected and the sample size appropriate for the study?*
5. Are the measurements used reliable and valid? *Are the data collection methods appropriate? Are all operational definitions clearly noted? Was a pilot study undertaken? How are reliability and validity determined?*
6. Is the data analysis described? *Is the data analysis appropriate for the study? Are any statistical tests clearly described? How are the results to be presented?*

Appraisal of the conduct of the research

1. Did the study proceed as intended? *If there were any alterations to the plan of the study, what effect did these have on the results?*
2. Were the findings described adequately? *Are the findings presented clearly and fully? Are any data missing or wrongly noted?*
3. Are all calculations correct? *Do the numbers add up? Were all tests performed correctly?*
4. Were the ethical considerations noted?

Assessing the outcomes of the research

1. What do the main findings mean? *Are the findings explained? Is the clinical significance of these findings stated?*

2. How are the hypotheses or research answers interpreted? *Have the hypotheses been proven? Are there any alternative explanations that can be given for the research findings?*
3. Are the conclusions justified? *Are they linked to the research aims and objectives? Are the conclusions reasonable based on your experience?*
4. How do the findings compare with what others have found? *Are they consistent with other findings? Are any differences from other studies discussed?*
5. How could you apply the findings to your clinical area? *Could the findings and conclusions apply to the clients in your clinical area? Do the benefits of these findings outweigh any potential risk or costs?*

SYSTEMATIC REVIEWS

Systematic reviews are analyses of research within a subject area that has already assessed in relation to its clinical effectiveness. There has been some criticism of systematic reviews in that the inclusion criteria for assessment are usually fairly stringent, with qualitative research being consistently overlooked. Crombie (1996) has identified the main issues that should be noted when assessing the quality of a systematic review (Box 8.2).

Box 8.2   *Appraisal questions for systematic reviews (Crombie 1996)*

- How were the research papers identified for reviewing?
- Is the subject area clearly defined?
- What exclusion criteria were applied?
- Was missing information sought?
- How was the quality of the papers assessed?
- Were the research designs noted in detail?
- How were the results summarized?
- Were differences in results investigated?
- Are there other findings which merit attention?

ETHICAL ISSUES

Mental health nurses have ethical responsibilities as part of their professional duty and ethical issues in research are now scrutinized quite closely. The RCN (1998) has published its own ethical guidelines in relation to research and the main principles are documented in Box 8.3.

Ethics committee

It is important to know that before any research can be undertaken, the researcher needs to obtain ethics committee approval for the study. Ethical committee approval should be gained for any research involving clients or health service staff, where the research is being carried out within health service premises or where the analysis and/or writing up of a research project is being done within health service premises. This can be a daunting process for any inexperienced nurse to undertake and you are strongly advised to get support from other nurses or health professionals who have taken proposals to an ethics committee. It is also helpful to seek the advice of any nurse member of the committee both to ensure that all the relevant information has been disclosed and also to gain an 'ally' in the committee. One final point of warning; it often takes three or more months to get from the point of initial contact to actually presenting a proposal to the ethics committee.

Box 8.3   RCN ethical guidelines

- Research must be necessary and contribute to further knowledge.
- Participants must receive full explanations of their involvement in the research and be told explicitly that they may refuse to participate.
- Consent must be obtained from the participant.
- Confidentiality must be maintained.
- The researcher must be qualified in the nature of the research problem and trained in appropriate research methods of design and analysis.
- Participants must be protected from pain, harm, injury and suffering.
- The relationship between the sponsor of the research and the researcher must be clearly stated.

THE RESEARCH PROPOSAL

On occasion, mental health nurses may have the opportunity to put forward research proposals in the attempt to gain funding or resources for a proposed study. The basic principles involved in doing this are documented below.

The actual content of the proposal may change depending on its nature and the reasons for its preparation. However, the following points should be considered.

1. Title of project
2. Summary
3. Justification for the study
4. Related research
5. Aims and objectives
6. Plan of investigation
7. Ethical considerations
8. Resources
9. Budget
10. Curriculum vitae

Title of project

Research projects become known by their title so it is important to make the title explicit and, while describing the proposed study, also make it relatively brief. The title should be able to override changes during the period of the study, whilst still being able to convey the essence of the research.

Summary

Most reward application bodies ask for a brief summary. In practice this is usually written after the main body of the proposal has been put together as it is a short statement about the objectives of the study and how it will be carried out.

Justification for the study

The statement of the problem, which opens up the proposal, must introduce the research questions and put them into a context which indicates the importance of the problem and the generalizability of the research. It should identify how the proposed study will build on previous work and add to theory.

Related research

It is important to demonstrate an appreciation of the current state of the topic area and the relevance of the planned study. A few key studies should be included which should relate to substantive concerns and to methods being proposed. Any knowledge of current research in the area may also be included.

Aims and objectives

The aims and objectives should be listed in order of importance and in a clear sequence. The remainder of the proposal will be judged on what the reader has been told about the aims of the study. Therefore the criteria need to be defined as specifically as possible. The objectives may take the form of questions, when research is exploratory, or a survey where specific facts are being sought. It may be possible to state objectives in the form of testable hypotheses where there is a basis for predicting results, such as in an experimental study.

Plan of investigation

The specific format will depend on the methods adopted. However, there are several important matters to convey and these are best written in discrete sections.

Population and sample

This will include the researcher's understanding of the numbers problem in relation to the amount of variability likely within the measures employed. It is better not to cut corners by suggesting smaller numbers than statistical analyses would demand, but limit numbers reasonably since more does not necessarily mean better quality. What is needed is evidence to show that the sample size is big enough to detect differences or will allow appropriate statistical manipulations to be carried out.

Particular sampling issues such as randomization will need to be explained. Convincing information needs to be supplied about the available sampling frame; in other words, the realistic sample population from which the research participants will be chosen. The description of the sample also needs to state the criteria for inclusion and exclusion, the recruitment issues and that consideration has been given to how non-respondents should be managed.

Design

The design will be a greater feature in experimental or survey research studies as it is clearly specifiable in advance. For experimental studies control groups, control of variables, randomization and matched groups will all need to be detailed. It is important to show an awareness of as many variables as possible and how control can be managed. The control of all variables is extremely difficult when conducting research on mental health issues. In survey designs, the proposal needs to show how the sample recruitment will occur and the expected numbers in the sample. It will also need to show how the study will manage a large number of respondents. In qualitative research, the design will be less specific but may include some details as to the types of approach that will be adopted by the researcher.

Data collection

The data collection instruments that are going to be used have to be stated. In certain cases (questionnaires, structured interviews) the collection technique is already established and a copy of the instrument should be sent with the proposal. If there is not a clearly established data collection tool, the principles behind the development of an instrument and procedures for establishing reliability and validity need to be stated. Within a qualitative study, the data collection techniques may be stated in general terms prior to the commencement of the study (e.g. unstructured interviews, observations, field notes). However, the data obtained can mean that the researcher will focus on a particular data collection method only after the study has commenced.

Data analysis

Finally, the proposed data analysis techniques should be documented.

WRITING UP A RESEARCH REPORT

Once a study has been finished, it is time to write the report. Even if the report is not destined for publication it is preferable to adopt the same format as for research articles in professional journals. Although different journals may have slightly different formats, the following is typical.

1. *Abstract* – a brief synopsis of the main rationale and findings of the study.

2. *Introduction* – what problem were you investigating and why?

3. *Literature review* – a guide to the current theories and research around the topic area(s).

4. *Method* – what procedures did you employ?

5. *Results* – what did you find?

6. *Discussion* – what do your findings mean?

7. *Conclusion* – a brief recounting of the main findings, and also where does the topic go from here?

8. *References* – an alphabetical list of books and articles cited in the report.

9. *Appendix* – this is optional, but would include copies of questionnaires, scales or stimulus materials used in the research or tables of data too extensive or too peripheral to include in the body of the report.

Introduction/literature review

The first task of the research report is to introduce the background and nature of the report being investigated.

To help the reader of the study, three rules apply.

1. Write in clear prose, not psychological or sociological jargon.

2. Don't plunge the unprepared reader into your problem or theory. Take the time necessary to lead up to the formal or theoretical statement bit by bit.

3. Use examples about theoretical points or to help introduce theoretical or technical terms.

After setting the stage with the opening statements, a summarization of the current state of knowledge in the area under investigation should be made. What previous research has been done with this problem? What are the relevant theories related to this phenomenon? The researcher should be familiar with previous work on the topic before embarking on the research design and therefore most of the literature search should be done by the time of writing the report. However, the results may have led to a reshaping of the study either by utilizing a different framework or by introducing a new aspect to the problem. New references might need to be found for these areas. It is unnecessary to cite every previous work published about a topic. Only cite articles that are pertinent to the issues being considered, emphasizing the major conclusions and findings or major methodological issues and avoiding excessive detail.

Method

The reader needs to know a considerable amount about the methodology used in the study. What was its basic design – experimental, survey, grounded theory, phenomenological? How were observations or variables translated into variables, e.g. how was caring assessed? The sample should be specified. Who were they? How were they chosen? How many? What procedures were adopted to collect the data? It is beneficial to label all the operations and variables with easy-to-remember names, e.g. the forensic group as opposed to the non-forensic group. Ethical considerations also need to be taken into account.

Results

In short articles these are sometimes combined with the discussion part of the report.

Two matters must be dealt with before presenting the main results.

There needs to be evidence that the study successfully set up the conditions for testing the hypotheses or answering the research questions. Were the people who participated in the study different from those who did not? If the study requires interrater judgement there should be evidence of interrater reliability. If certain subjects had to be discarded the effect on the results should be mentioned. Some of these issues may be discussed in the methods section.

The method of data analysis. Initially this will involve describing the main procedures in converting raw observations into analysable data. Again, these may be included in the methods section. Following on from this should be a description of the statistical analysis itself. If it is a standard test, this can be briefly described. If it is unconventional, it may require a rationale, preferably supported by published evidence.

The findings

The main point to remember is to begin with the central findings and then move on to the peripheral ones.

1. Remind the reader of the conceptual question, e.g. medium secure units are less violent than inner-city generic wards.
2. Remind the reader of the operational statement which is the operation or behaviour measured, e.g. the amount of staff physically assaulted in inner-city wards is higher than in medium secure units.
3. Give the answer: yes/no.
4. Follow this up with the statistical evidence.
5. Any elaboration or qualification can then be made, e.g. only in one MSU were there generally more assaults on staff.
6. Every finding that involves a comparison between groups or relationships between variables should be accompanied by its level of statistical significance.
7. In selecting descriptive indices or statistics, the purpose is to be as descriptive of the actual behaviours observed as possible.
8. In qualitative research, statistical tests are rarely performed yet the reader needs to be informed of the relationships between different variables; this is usually done in either a textual or figurative manner.
9. Every set of findings that are sufficiently important to be stressed should be accompanied by a table, graph or figure showing the relevant data. The basic rule here is that readers should be able to grasp the main points either by reading the text or by looking at the figures and tables.
10. End each section of the results with a summary of the main point raised.

Discussion

The discussion forms a narrative with the introduction and it may be necessary to move materials back and forth between the introduction and discussion as the report is redeveloped. Topics that are central to the argument will appear in the introduction and possibly again in the discussion. Points that are less important may be left until the discussion phase.

It is helpful to initially identify what has been learned from the study. This should include a clear statement in support or denial of the hypotheses or the answers to the questions raised in the introduction. It should not be a reformulation of the results but should contribute something new to the reader's understanding of the problem, including what inferences can be drawn from the findings. Comparisons with other findings may also be appropriate. This may include identifying shortcomings in your study or conditions that may limit generalization of the study. It is important that researchers are willing to accept negative or unexpected results.

The discussion should also include an overview of the questions that remain unanswered or new questions that have been raised by the study along with suggestions for the kinds of research that would help to answer them.

Summary/conclusion

This is a very brief summary that restates, in barest outline, the problem, the procedures, the major findings and the major conclusions drawn from them.

References

All books and articles cited in the text of a report are listed at the end using a valid referencing system such as the Harvard or Vancouver referencing system. Different publications and different institutions have their own preferences as to which is preferred.

Appendix

The appendix of a report contains copies of materials used in the study that would be too expensive to include in the report itself. This might include questionnaires, attitude scales, stimulus materials and photographs and would assist other researchers replicating the study. Tables of data or additional table analyses that are too extensive or peripheral to include in the report itself allow an interested reader to explore the data in fine detail or to answer questions about the results. Most journals have minimal appendices due to limited space but appendices are common in academic work.

AREAS FOR POTENTIAL RESEARCH

One of the main difficulties when mental health nurses start thinking about research is in relation to the focus of any research study. In general terms, if nurses find difficulty in obtaining consistent information about an area or they have some existing knowledge or enthusiasm, these could both be the starting point for undertaking a research project. However, certain specific areas of research will have more relevance to mental health nurses in general as they may focus on topical issues. They will also be more likely to attract funding from outside agencies.

The Mental Health National Service Frameworks (NHSE 1999b) provide guidance on six areas where national standards of care should be provided. These are the mental health issues that should be given priority in the development of services within the five years following the report. The areas are:

- mental health promotion
- primary care
- access to services
- effective service for people with severe mental illness
- caring about carers
- preventing suicide.

CONCLUSION

Mental health nurses involved in research need to have a clear understanding of the research process and to be able to use this knowledge in the development of research proposals. It is also important that mental health nurses are able to present the results of their research to a wider audience either through submissions to journals, publishing on the Internet or though conference presentations. Some areas for future mental health nursing research have been suggested within the chapter where there is the opportunity for joint research with other disciplines and where financial assistance could be available.

Mental health nursing is an increasingly complex and evolving discipline which needs to use research to extend its knowledge base and prove its clinical effectiveness over the coming years. The ability to engage in research projects, either on an individual basis or as part of a group, will lead the profession to focus more clearly on its role and its development in the years to come.

REFERENCES

Brooker, C., Falloon, I., Butterworth, A. *et al.* (1994) The outcome of training community psychiatric nurses to deliver psychosocial intervention. *British Journal of Psychiatry* 165: 222–230.

Burns, N. and Grove, S. (1993) *The Practice of Nursing Research: conduct, critique and utilization.* W.B. Saunders, Philadelphia.

Carpenter, W., Buchanan, R., Kirkpatrick, B. *et al.* (1999) Comparative effectiveness of fluphenazine decanoate injections every 2 weeks versus every 6 weeks. *American Journal of Psychiatry* 156(3): 412–418.

Cormack, D. (1996) *The Research Process in Nursing.* Blackwell, London.

Crombie, K. (1996) *The Pocket Guide to Critical Appraisal.* BMJ Publishing Group, London.

Cullum, N. (1998) Evidence-Based Practice. *Nursing Management* 5(3): 32–35.

Hek, G., Judd, M. and Moule, P. (1996) *Making Sense of Research: an introduction for nurses.* Cassell, London.

Lepola, I. and Vanhanen, L. (1997) The patient's daily activities in psychiatric care. *Journal of Psychiatric and Mental Health Nursing* 4(1): 29–36.

MacInnes, D. (1998) The differences between health professionals in assessing levels of caregiver burden. *Journal of Psychiatric and Mental Health Nursing* 5(4): 265–272.

MacLeod-Clark, J. and Hockey, L. (1989) *Further Research for Nursing.* Scutari Press, London.

NHSE (1997) *Promoting Clinical Effectiveness: a framework for action in and through the NHS.* Department of Health, London.

NHSE (1999a) *Achieving Effective Practice.* Department of Health, London.

NHSE (1999b) *Modern Standards and Service Models: mental health national service frameworks.* Department of Health, London.

Parahoo, K. (1997) *Nursing Research: principles, processes and issues.* Macmillan, London.

Parahoo, K. (1999) A comparison of pre-Project 2000 and Project 2000 nurses' perceptions of their research training, research needs and of their use of research in clinical areas. *Journal of Advanced Nursing* 29(1): 237–245.

Polit, D. and Hungler, B. (1993) *Essentials of Nursing Research.* Lippincott, Philadelphia.

RCN (1998) *Research Ethics: guidance for nurses involved in research or any investigative project involving human subjects.* RCN, London.

Robson, C. (1997) *Real World Research.* Blackwell, Oxford.

SNMAC (1999) *Mental Health Nursing: addressing acute concerns.* Department of Health, London.

UKCC (1996) *Code of Professional Conduct for the Nurse, Midwife and Health Visitor.* UKCC, London.

WENR (2000) Proceedings of the 10th biennial conference – Challenges for Nurses in the 21st Century: Health Promotion, Prevention and Intervention. WENR, Reykjavik.

White, E. (1990) *The Third Quinquennial Survey of Community Psychiatric Services.* Department of Nursing, University of Manchester.

Yonge, O., Qiupling, Z. and Zelski, J. (1997) Variables and designs in psychiatric/mental health nursing research articles published from 1982 to 1992. *Journal of Psychiatric and Mental Health Nursing* 4(4): 339–343.

9 THE NURSE AS CLINICIAN

Sheila Forster, Matthew Morrissey and Mark Wilbourn

OBJECTIVES

After reading this chapter, you should be able to:

- understand the basic nursing skills required by nurses working in different settings
- critically evaluate your own skills in similar situations.

INTRODUCTION

It will be evident from reading preceding chapters that mental health nursing is considered to be a dynamic, creative, therapeutic relationship with clients. As such, it is dependent upon the nurse employing research, reflection and evidence-based practice as the 'knowledgeable doer'.

For many years (see Chapter 1), the actual task of mental health nursing was seen as just that – a set of tasks which were commonly carried out in a mechanistic way. Once the sequence of events and the equipment required had been memorized, the procedure was dutifully carried out, more or less efficiently but with minimal thought attached to it; a legacy of the doctor's handmaiden role which has dogged nursing for so many years (Cormack 1983, Towell 1975).

Emphasis on procedure and tasks not only dominated day-to-day practice but was the basis for nurse training. Until the advent of the 1982 syllabus of training for mental nurses, previous syllabuses required that a schedule of practical experiences had to be completed during the three-year period. This schedule comprised lists of situations, tasks and procedures that nurses were likely to encounter and therefore needed to demonstrate some degree of proficiency in dealing with them efficiently.

The focus of this schedule was very much on physical tasks such as 'nursing the bedridden patient', 'dealing with epileptic seizures' and 'administering first aid'. Administrative procedures were also to the fore to ensure that the ordering, monitoring and storage of drugs, food, clothing, toiletries etc. were well rehearsed. Sadly, little emphasis was placed on what we now consider to be the prime skills of the mental health nurse, communication and interpersonal relationships, and the most complicated piece of equipment that a mental health nurse employed on a daily basis, namely their personality, was barely mentioned.

With hindsight, it is easy to criticize these early attempts to ensure that mental health nurses were 'properly trained'. However, the importance of many of these tasks and the practical skills required to carry them out effectively should not be underestimated; they were and still are essential to the provision of holistic care.

It is the intention of this chapter to identify, consider and discuss the responsibilities of the mental health nurse in relation to practical skills, physical treatments and psychological therapies, whilst not losing sight of the need to constantly evaluate, reflect upon and apply theory to practice, thus preventing the application of skilled nursing care being reduced yet again to a set of tasks and procedures. However, to achieve this aim whilst at the same time maintaining clarity for the reader, a 'shopping list' type format of the core skills, not dissimilar to the old-fashioned schedule referred to above, has been employed. Readers are implored to constantly bear in mind that the points, principles and suggestions contained in this chapter *must* be adapted to accurately meet the needs of each individual in their care.

In this chapter we have looked at the four most common areas in which mental health nurses work: working in the community, acute inpatient care, rehabilitation and care of the elderly, since these areas are where most mental health nurses begin their careers. We recognize that there are also many specialist areas, such as working with children and families, but the intention of this chapter is to demonstrate the basic 'building blocks' that are needed by all mental health nurses before going into more specialist careers, such as are described in *Working in Partnership* (DoH 1994, Annexe F). Each section therefore looks at the basic clinical areas and provides examples of clients who may be encountered and the skills that can be used by the nurse in that setting.

WORKING IN THE COMMUNITY

Val Hayton works with the community mental health team that is based on the site of a GP-run hospital in a small seaside town. There are three other CPNs in the team, plus an occupational therapist. The nearest inpatient facilities are 35 miles away, where Val attends a ward round each week, and there is a day services unit in the next town eight miles away. The average caseload size is 38, which is generic. There is a community assessment team for the elderly based at the day centre, a child and family community team in the same town and a team working with substance abusers. Referrals come mainly from the four GP practices in the town but also from the psychiatrist, families and self-referrals. It is aimed to see urgent referrals within 24 hours for those who have, for example, taken unplanned discharge from hospital and have no social support and are deemed vulnerable.

In this section, the two main areas of Val's work will be looked at to identify the skills that are used: working with those who require long-term care and short-term contacts with the acutely ill.

Working with those who require long-term care

Matthew James is 28 and was admitted to the acute admission ward six weeks ago, following a GP visit to his house at the request of his mother with whom he lives. She is widowed and Matthew lives alone with her. He has not worked since leaving school and has few social contacts, spending most of his time playing computer games.

Over the past few weeks his conversation had become increasingly strange and he told his mother that he was the wizard in the game and that he could make things happen to people if he didn't like them. His behaviour towards her became increasingly hostile and he refused to eat anything that she had cooked because he said she didn't want him alive any more. She finally called the GP when he barricaded himself in his room and Val accompanied the GP on this visit and persuaded Matthew to come into hospital. He was prescribed haloperidol on admission, which seems to have reduced his suspicious behaviour and will be prescribed clopixol prior to discharge. His mother has been told that he will be able to come home next week, which she is not happy about. She is of the strong opinion that he will become ill as soon as he comes home again and that he should stay in hospital for much longer, even though it has been explained to her that his symptoms are under control now and he needs to be at home trying to make a new life.

The families of the long-term mentally ill are those most likely to provide the care and support necessary for living in the community. As this was Matthew's first admission, it is clear that there will need to be a strong supportive relationship between Matthews, his mother and the CPN. Winefield and Harvey (1994) surveyed 121 carers of those with long-term mental health problems and found that their main stated needs were as follows:

- support
- less social isolation
- to know that there are others in the same situation
- information about the illness and treatment
- advice about coping strategies
- familiarity with mental health resources.

The CPN in this situation must therefore develop a trusting relationship with both Matthew and his mother, if possible starting before discharge, since this will help to reduce the apprehension that she will inevitably feel at the thought of the future. Val will need to check out what his mother actually knows about his illness and gently find out what fears she has about him coming home. It could be wrongly assumed that just because he is her son, she welcomes him coming home. She may well feel frightened or even not want him to come home, depending on her knowledge of how he may behave in future. Encouraging a supportive atmosphere significantly reduces relapse rates (Gamble 1993) and so Val needs to work with his mother on ways of giving Matthew support, by encouraging positive behaviour.

Falloon (1984) devised a simple behavioural social skills training for families caring for those with mental health problems. For example, if wishing to encourage positive feelings towards each other the following steps can be taken.

- Look at the person.
- Say exactly what they did that pleased you.
- Tell them how it made you feel.

In this way the behaviour that the carer wants is reinforced although as Matthew's mother has not used this technique before, Val will need to work with her to reinforce it.

Finally, Mrs James will need a variety of informative interventions. How can she contact Val should she need to? What resources and agencies are available both for her and Matthew? Is there a carer's group in the town? What should she look out for that would suggest that Matthew is becoming unwell again? Val will need to spend a lot of time answering these and other questions that will help Mrs James to feel less isolated and reduce any fears that she may have about not being able to cope.

Matthew himself will also be seen regularly by Val. He is likely to be very suspicious of her at first, particularly if he feels that she and his mother are colluding in a conspiracy against him. The transition from hospital to home may feel frightening, since his admission from home when he was very unwell will be remembered. Segal (1991) states that 'desperate unhappiness and longing may be encountered along with cruelty, perversity, blame and rejection (p. 107). Val's focus with Matthew is to discover ways of enabling him to live not just with his illness, but also with his environment. How much does he know about his illness? Does he understand why the medication he has been prescribed is so important and how can he change the pattern of his life so that he does not drift back into isolation?

Working with people with an enduring mental illness presents significant challenges for mental health nurses. Progress may be slow and the client may have little motivation. Val may choose to use psychosocial interventions in tandem with Matthew's mother.

It will be obvious to Val that Matthew's mother cannot be expected to provide total care for Matthew and that he will need help to look after himself. Social skills training, described by Libermann (1992) as 'behavioural techniques or learning activities that enable people to establish or restore instrumental or affiliate skills in domains required to meet the interpersonal, self care and coping demands of community living' (p. 94) will probably be useful. Val should therefore establish with Matthew what his daily life was like before he became ill and what his level of functioning is in social skills terms. For example, how capable was he of looking after himself then and what does he need to learn to look after himself now? The local resource house can play an important part here. It is used regularly by up to 14 users of mental health services and provides a safe environment where social activities take place and basic living skills can be practised, with the more expert teaching the less expert. He will also have access to equipment that he can use and then repeat at home. There is also the advantage that Matthew will start to meet new people at the house, some of whom will have had the same experiences as him.

Close monitoring of his medication is also an important factor.

Short-term contacts with the acutely ill

Jane Brown, aged 36, has been referred to the CPN team by her GP. She had a miscarriage a year ago and has been unable to conceive since. She began having panic attacks a few months after the miscarriage which became worse when she left the house. She now feels unable to go out and suffers from frequent panic attacks with accompanying hyperventilation. She complains of insomnia, loss of appetite and frequent attacks of crying. She is unwilling to take any medication but says she will do 'anything to be able to go out again'. Her husband Peter, is keen to help but is away from home during the week, working. They are both regular churchgoers and have a wide circle of friends there. Jane is particularly concerned about the effects of her illness on her marriage, since she is finding it increasingly difficult to relate with any warmth to Peter and frequently loses her temper with him over trivial things, resulting in him leaving the house in a temper.

Jackman (1992) studied mothers who had lost their babies and found that 44% were still experiencing notable psychological distress a year after the loss and Val will be aware that the symptoms Jane is experiencing are part of the loss process. Much will depend on Val's ability to reassure Jane that these symptoms are not uncommon or unnatural. Stewart (1994) states that 'pregnancy changes the role from an individual to a creator and nurturer, bringing with it a whole range of hopes, fears and dreams' (p. 15). The loss of this role brings with it 'a huge human loss and weight of sadness' and the way that Jane was treated after her miscarriage may have influenced the way she feels now.

Val's role is to work with Jane on several issues. First, she needs to go back to the loss with Jane, using her counselling skills, which may entail recreating memories of what happened and checking that they have been fully acknowledged (Sherr 1995). Jane may have photographs or clothes that were bought for the baby and looking at these together will induce a cathartic response which may be very useful. Heron (1997) points out that because catharsis is such a powerful release of emotion, the client needs to 'give permission' for this to take place, since at its deepest level, the release of fear, grief or anger needs to be prepared for. If this is not done, or was not done fully at the time, then the grieving process is hampered and results in the type of psychological symptoms that Jane is experiencing.

Second, the link between grief and distress needs to be fully comprehended by Jane, so that she can understand why she is reacting as she is. Her relationship with her husband has inevitably been affected and following miscarriage this is common, since on the one hand, the mother feels anger, guilt and loss of self-esteem, which affects the relationship, and on the other, the husband often feels left out of the grief and unable to express his feelings as fully as the mother (Stewart 1994). Finally, Val will need to address the anxiety and panic attacks and undertake a behavioural programme, together with relaxation work, which will help Jane to resume a normal life.

Working with Jane will be facilitated by using a contract, agreeing together on how many sessions they need to have and involving her husband and friends as appropriate during the week when they are unable to meet. Jane should be asked initially to keep a diary in which to note down when she feels worst and what is happening at the time, to give Val some idea of the 'early warning signs' which indicate the onset of panic (Keable 1989). Jane also needs to know how to control the panic, using relaxation techniques which she can practise daily. Hyperventilation can often be helped by breathing into cupped hands or into a paper bag. It is very important that Jane understands the full effects of anxiety on the body as then the symptoms should become less frightening. Friends can also be encouraged to take part in gradual exposure to going outside. Val can start this process by asking Jane to make a list of all the frightening things that she can think of and then list these in order of importance so that together they can plan a gentle exposure to frightening stimuli over the weeks of the contract. Her husband and friends whom she trusts can then help her in this exposure.

Ash (1997) suggests a 'funnelling format' that can be used to identify for Jane exactly what the problem behaviour is and what makes it better or worse. Once this has been established, Val can then work with Jane on the formulation of goal statements which include realistic expectations and achievements, however small they may seem; for example, 'I will walk to church with Peter on Sundays and stay for the first part of the service'.

However, as her husband works away from home during the week, it may be appropriate for Val to suggest to Jane that she attends the local day centre to take part in anxiety management groups, including relaxation experience. Local groups run by the Miscarriage Association or the Stillbirth and Neonatal Society can also be contacted to provide not only information resources but also befriending, as it may be of particular value to Jane to talk to other women who can share her experience.

It can be seen that the work Val does with Jane is quite different from that with Matthew and his mother, employing skills of support and behavioural techniques, in addition to providing access to specific facilities that will reinforce the work done by Jane and her husband.

WORKING IN AN ACUTE INPATIENT SETTING

Health-care legislation, including the introduction on 1 April 1996 of the new arrangements for aftercare under supervision in the form of a process of supervised discharge (NHSE 1996), emphasized the need to care for people in the community wherever possible. However, there are times when individuals require care in hospital. Care for many mentally ill people during the most acute phases of their illness takes place on psychiatric wards. Nursing staff working in these areas must have many skills to be able to deliver high-quality care in what is a highly stressful work environment. Society is changing and the effects of stressful living and drugs become ever more apparent on the ward.

This section of the chapter examines the skills required of the nurse working in an inpatient setting. These are discussed in relation to the interpersonal nursing theory of Hildegard Peplau (1952) who describes nursing as a significant therapeutic interpersonal process in which both parties grow as a result of channelling the energy created in stress. The model of care aims to identify interpersonal problems and encourage attempts at more successful styles of relating (Cutting 1997). It is both purposeful and goal centred with the nurse helping to channel the patient's energy towards interpersonal growth. Through this process the nurse adopts many roles including that of stranger, teacher, leader, counsellor, resource person and surrogate. Peplau's model of care consists of four phases in which the nurse and patient play an active role:

- orientation
- identification
- exploitation
- resolution.

Paul is a staff nurse working on an acute mental health unit. he has been qualified for a couple of years during which time he has worked exclusively with adult inpatients. The ward on which he works has 15 beds providing inpatient care for a local urban population. The team is made up of nurses, a consultant psychiatrist and his senior house officer and part-time input from an occupational therapist. Close working relationships are maintained with the community mental health team and other external agencies. Reference will be made to common disorders affecting thought, perception and mood to highlight the skills employed by Paul in working with Peplau's model.

Orientation phase

The first stage of Peplau's model, the orientation phase, gives Paul an opportunity to build a relationship with his patients, gaining their trust and forming the basis on which they will work together. Paul must demonstrate empathy, genuineness, warmth and understanding. This responses should be positive and without judgement or conditions. He must also be aware of his own values, beliefs and prejudices, particularly when dealing with patients who have conflicting values and beliefs. Nurses often have strong views about people who abuse alcohol, for instance, and should be conscious of not allowing their rigid value systems to reduce the likelihood of developing empathic, caring relationships. Through demonstrating respect for his patients, Paul begins to build trust within the relationship that will form the basis of future care. The nurse must be able to communicate effectively with patients at all levels (Hargie 1997). An open posture and demonstrating active listening will help Paul to establish rapport. Sensitivity to non-verbal communication will help him in his assessment of the mental state of the patient.

Paul has recently assessed a patient, Rob, who was responding to auditory hallucinations, and expressing bizarre delusional thoughts about alien invasions and transmitters in his brain. Rob believed that he could receive messages through the television screen that no-one else was able to interpret. He was often observed to be laughing, smiling and grimacing, which was out of context for the conversation. This is a good indication that Rob is hallucinating. Reflecting on and summarizing important points and the use of verbal and non-verbal prompts will help to keep Rob focused on the conversation; hallucinations can be distracting to the patient. The patient may also develop a language of their own or express bizarre ideas or resist the nurses attempts to communicate and direct anger towards them. The nurse must acknowledge the perceptions and feelings of the patient and work with them in developing the relationship. This can be enhanced through maintaining eye contact, appropriate use of touch and adopting an open posture. When a patient is expressing delusional beliefs, as is the case with Rob, the nurse may find it useful to work with the feelings rather than the thoughts or ideas that form the delusion. This helps to avoid confrontation over the validity of the beliefs.

Identification phase

The next phase involves the identification if problems and setting of goals (Nelson-Jones 1993). This is an interpersonal process between the nurse, patient and carers. Skills of observation and effective communication help the nurse to assess the problems experienced by the patient and identify their needs. This is a continual process of establishing what is normal for the patient and ensuring that the setting of goals is appropriate. It is also important for the nurse to prioritize needs through the setting of both short- and long-term goals. Short-term goals can be seen to be within reach by the patient and progress will reinforce a belief that longer term goals can be achieved. It is essential that the goals made are realistic and achievable.

A hierarchy of needs (Maslow 1962) exists for patients and should be considered during the identification phase. Basic needs must be met before a patient can move towards higher needs. Paul identified a short-term goal of rehydration for a depressed patient who has stopped eating and drinking whereas in caring for an overactive or suicidal patient, he will need to consider safety as a priority. Paul must have an awareness of high-risk factors such as those associated with suicide. These include the presence of mental and physical illness, previous suicide attempts, low self-esteem, bizarre ideation and the influence of alcohol and drugs. The plan of care identified for the patient will reflect the relative safety concerns and will seek to maintain a safe environment.

Many patients are aggressive when confronted with a stay in hospital. Paul has been working with Adam, who has a long history of both verbal and physical aggression when confined by a claustrophobic ward environment. This aggression normally centres on an inability to communicate effectively emotional, physical or interpersonal problems. When confronted by aggression, Paul has a responsibility to himself, his colleagues and Adam to promote the safety of all concerned. This entails having in place appropriate management plans and a consistent approach from staff. Paul must be aware of the short-term needs of the patient, which may include safety and security, autonomy, space, comfort and understanding. This can be achieved with sensitive communication although there are times when physical intervention is appropriate for the safety of those in the immediate environment.

For many patients attaining long-term goals can be a very slow process. Joanne has been in hospital on numerous occasions, usually following an overdose precipitated by an argument with her husband. Despite no obvious depressive illness Joanne is usually able to secure an admission to the ward at these times. Manipulative patients like Joanne often have an emotional deficit, which presents as learned maladaptive behaviour. Exaggerated claims of overdoses and engineering longer stays in hospital can be extremely frustrating for nursing staff. The danger is that such behaviour can lead to alienation of nursing staff for patients that require considerable input. Paul must demonstrate acceptable behaviour by showing warmth and honesty. Consistent communication and approach will reinforce appropriate behaviour while inconsistency can lead to further manipulation. Attention may be sought through suicidal gestures, aggression and antisocial behaviour. Learning acceptable behaviour patterns and becoming more trusting, warm and honest is often a protracted and frustrating experience for the nurse. It is important at the identification phase for Paul to discuss in a caring way the inappropriateness of the behaviour, explore reasons for the behaviour and set limits on the behaviour. Paul will act as a role model to the patient in this process.

Exploitation phase

The third phase, exploitation, is the time when the plan of care is implemented – the working phase of the model. During this phase the therapeutic relationship formed with the nurse enables the patient to move forward or grow (Forster 1997).

It is important for the nurse to have a sound understanding of the effects that mental disorders can have on individuals (Janosik 1996). Features of psychosis, for example, are not amenable to suggestion and should be recognized as such. Negative symptoms can be confused with intentional stubborn behaviour and antipsychotic drugs can exacerbate these. Understanding the biological and pharmacological bases to the behaviour will help the nurse with interpretation and inform their practice. The nurse must have an understanding of the impact of stressful interactions on the mental state of the patients in their care, such as isolation and loneliness and fear of the future. Stress increases the severity of symptoms. The role of the nurse is to promote a reduction in the level of stress in the patient and help improve their coping skills. This should be achieved through working with the family/carers wherever possible, educating them about the illness and the influence of stressful situations and factors such as drug misuse and poor compliance with prescribed medications. These should all be elicited alongside basic needs such as adequate housing and employment and recreational opportunities.

Paul is working with the family of a young woman who has recently experienced her first psychotic episode. Jenny became unwell when she started to attend university. She is very bright, as are her two sisters. The family all work in the field of law, and Jenny, the youngest, is expected to follow the same path. Paul is offering guidance to the parents about possible contributory factors to their daughter's illness and ways to promote future well-being. He explains to them the impact that stressful situations, such as the expectations of achieving in a very competitive field, can have on an individual and ways of reducing or coping with them. His work with Jenny also addresses these issues and highlights the need to take advantage of the support around her, both from her family and professionals.

Patients in acute phases of mental illness often exhibit disorders of thought and perception (Barker 1997). Paranoid patients, perceiving a threat, require sensitivity at a time when they are feeling particularly vulnerable. Preoccupation with delusional ideas can hinder the attempts of the nurse to communicate with the patient. The nurse must allow the patient to ventilate their concerns whilst being cautious not to collude with the ideas being expressed. Liam has been a patient in the ward for several weeks. He was admitted following a relapse of a paranoid illness. He believes a secret agent is attempting to harm him for something he did a long time ago. The trust and understanding developing between Paul and Liam during the orientation and identification phases offer greater opportunity for Paul to distract Liam from his thoughts. The way Paul communicates should be open and reassuring with appropriate behaviour being encouraged and rewarded. Paul avoids overuse of touch as Liam perceives this to be threatening.

Many of these skills are similar to those used with patients who are hallucinating. The nurse must deny sharing the experiences of the patient without arguing about validity or appearing to make judgements. It is important that the nurse acknowledges the contribution that the hallucinations make to the way the patient is feeling and avoids trivializing their experience. Antipsychotic drugs can provide much relief for patients with disorders of thought and perception. It is important that any medication is offered with gentle encouragement; being overpersuasive can be damaging to the relationship. There are times when the use of intramuscular medication is beneficial to the patient as it can be administered quickly and avoids potentially harmful protracted discussions.

Patients with disorders of mood form a significant proportion of the psychiatric ward population. Mood can be depressed or elated and accompanied by psychosocial and behavioural problems. These are often the focus of nursing interventions and are supported by the therapeutic relationship. Paul has a role in educating patients about their illness and treatments, supporting them in dealing with conflict and stress and helping them to realize their potential. Shirley is experiencing low mood consequential to bereavement. Her husband died unexpectedly just before their wedding anniversary. In this instance Paul must be sensitive to the grieving process and aware of the difficulties this can present. Outpourings of emotion, including anger and resentment, must be met by a caring empathic nurse who is able to absorb the interpersonal exchanges and continue to be supportive.

Pharmacological treatment of depression tends to involve the use of antidepressants such as serotonin reuptake inhibitors (SSRIs), tricyclic antidepressants (TCAs) and monoamine oxidase inhibitors (MAOIs), with lithium sometimes being used as an adjunct. There is generally an early improvement in most symptoms of depressive illness when antidepressants are used although cognitive symptoms such as low self-esteem tend to respond slowly; a delayed response of 3–4 weeks is normal. There are circumstances when electroconvulsive therapy (ECT) can be used for the treatment of depressed mood; refractory depression and depression in frail older people are two examples.

The elated, overactive patient often behaves in an unpredictable way that compromises their safety or dignity. Lucy was admitted to the ward having been stopped by the police for dangerous and erratic driving. Since this time she has been very demonstrative and often disinhibited in her behaviour. Creating an environment with minimal stimulation is often the best immediate response to limiting this behaviour and ensuring that both her safety and dignity are maintained. Communication by means of gentle, persuasion and suggestion can be a more productive approach when dealing with unpredictable behaviour. This may aver confrontation. However, there are times when no matter how Paul attempts to communicate with Lucy she still reacts to confinement by becoming aggressive. The trust developed between Paul and Lucy during the first two phases of Peplau's model promotes greater understanding between them at this stage (Wykes 1993). Paul is more able to absorb the hostility whilst continuing to model calm, appropriate behaviour. Distraction, reassurance and setting of limits on behaviour can all be effective interventions.

Medication is also often used to complement nursing interventions, particularly when the patient is acutely disturbed. Antipsychotic drugs are given to redress neurotransmitter imbalances in the dopamine system. They have the potential to counteract the underlying neurochemical basis of the illness whilst offering some welcome sedative response. Antipsychotic drugs are often used in conjunction with short-acting benzodiazepines to promote a speedy return to a level of tranquillity. This can be of enormous help in maintaining the safety of the patient and those around. It is important that Paul gives Lucy every opportunity to accept the medication freely, offering it in the most acceptable form with a full explanation for the reasons it is being given and the potential benefits. If medication is given without the consent of the patient, as is sometimes necessary, future compliance with other treatments may be compromised.

When the mood of a patient cycles from elation to depression, as is the case with bipolar illness, lithium is often used to add stability. The mode of action of lithium and other mood-stabilizing drugs is unclear but the nurse should ensure that the patient is fully aware of the need to take the drug as prescribed and to attend for monitoring of blood serum levels. The nurse should also be aware of the signs and symptoms of lithium toxicity and protocols for dealing with this.

The care of individuals with a dual diagnosis is becoming an ever-increasing problem on psychiatric wards (Boyd and Bihart 1998). Part of the difficulty in providing care arises from confusion about whether the symptoms are precipitated by a mental disorder or are the effects of substances used by the patient. There is also the possibility that the use of substances is an attempt by the patient to mask the effects of the underlying illness. Nevertheless the high incidence of dually diagnosed individuals provides a further dimension to the work of the mental health nurse.

It is not uncommon for patients to be admitted to psychiatric wards for detoxification from alcohol. The treatment involves restoring homeostasis for the patient, by providing them with nutrition and security. Fred was admitted to the ward following several unsuccessful attempts at home detoxification. During the admission he showed significant withdrawal symptoms, indicating the need for medication to provide some relief. Paul administered a long-acting benzodiazepine, chlordiazepoxide, in gradually reducing doses, making the whole process safer and more tolerable for Fred. The nurse must be aware of potential problems such as increased likelihood of fits and delirium tremens. Longer term pharmacological treatments often involve prophylactics such a disulfirum, given in tandem with support for emotional, social and financial problems.

Resolution phase

The final phase of Peplau's developmental model, resolution, is where the nurse–patient relationship draws to a conclusion. It is a time when the patient moves towards regaining their independence and the nurse evaluates the interpersonal processes that have led to growth for both the patient and the nurse. Paul prepares his patients for the resolution phase from the time of their admission to hospital. This phase can then be used to clarify discharge arrangements with appropriate parties, including carers, friends and relatives, and professional support such as that provided by community mental health teams.

The needs addressed in the resolution phase will be specific to the patient. However, it is likely that people like Rob, Jenny, Liam and Lucy will require some form of follow-up from the community mental health team who will monitor their progress and ensure that their basic needs, such as finance and housing, are met. The support required by Shirley is likely to be short term and will come mainly from family and friends whilst Fred may be seen by a member of the alcohol team who will work closely with his general practitioner. The post-discharge plans for Joanne will enable a consistent approach from all those involved in her care in order to effectively manage likely disruptive behaviour in the future.

WORKING IN REHABILITATION SETTINGS

Martin is a deputy manager (F grade) in a 10-bedded rehabilitation unit. He has worked at the unit since it opened two years ago. At the present time there are nine patients, four men and five women, most of whom joined the unit at the same time as Martin.

The clinical skills that Martin employs can be identified and discussed under the activities of living as outlined by Roper *et al.* (1996):

- maintaining a safe environment
- breathing
- communicating
- eating and drinking
- eliminating
- personal cleansing and dressing
- controlling body temperature
- mobilizing
- working and playing
- expressing sexuality
- sleeping
- dying.

Maintaining a safe environment

Martin is aware that all the patients in his care have some degree of impairment in relation to the recognition of environmental risk factors. Therefore, he uses his observation skills to minimize the risks to the patients and assists them to recognize, reduce, and avoid harmful situations and behaviours.

For example, Harry, who is 52 years old, has spent much of his adult life in a variety of wards in a large psychiatric hospital. As a consequence of this, he displays signs of institutionalization. This, coupled with his enduring mental health problem (schizophrenia), compromises Harry's safety in two particular areas. First, Harry is a heavy smoker who likes to smoke in bed. Martin has to use his sense of smell and sight to monitor Harry's behaviour and reduce the risk of fire. Second, Harry's reduced environmental awareness is made worse because he has a hearing impairment. This puts him greatly at risk when he leaves the unit to go to the local village. Martin has to ensure that he is accompanied so that he can be helped to practise sound roadcraft skills and thus avoid traffic accidents.

Breathing

In common with Harry, most of the patients are quite heavy smokers. Martin is very aware of how smoking can have detrimental effects on health. He therefore monitors the amount that each person smokes and observes them for shortness of breath, wheezing, coughing and expectorating. He is even more vigilant in the winter months because three patients suffer from chronic bronchitis and are prone to recurrent chest infections. Martin must be skilled in recognizing the early signs of chest infection, organize a medical assessment, ensure that any prescribed treatment is accurately administered and be familiar with and observe for therapeutic and unwanted effects.

Communicating

Due to the effects of severe and enduring mental illness, the majority of Martin's patients experience some difficulty in communicating effectively. Molly, for example, finds it very difficult to relate to others. She tends to avoid social contact and displays disordered thinking in her conversational content, often resorting to her own private language which is littered with neologisms (new words) and expletives. Martin, aware that this behaviour makes it difficult for Molly to be accepted readily by the local community, tries to help her to convey her thoughts, feelings, wants and needs in a more coherent, socially acceptable manner. This requires Martin to use active listening, sensitive responding and accurate interpretation skills to assist Molly to express herself more clearly and ensure that her needs are understood so that they can be met.

A similar situation arises with Jean, who expresses physical concerns in tangential, indirect ways. Again, Martin needs to be constantly aware of Jean's idiosyncrasies and be able to accurately identify what she is trying to convey. For example, he has learned that when Jean angrily tells others that 'the devil has got his arm half way down my throat and is biting my bum', it means that she has become constipated and is experiencing haemorrhoidal pain. As with Molly, Martin has to be very tactful and diplomatic when working with Jean so that he does not embarrass or offend her as he helps her to find alternative ways of expressing her physical ailments.

Eating and drinking

All the patients are encouraged to be involved in the choice, purchase and preparation of food. Martin needs to monitor these activities and, recognizing that decision making, budgeting and cooking skills are very challenging for a number of the patients, decide on the level of support and assistance he will offer. He sometimes feels that it would be much easier all round if the nursing team carried out these activities *for* rather than *with* the patients but he resists the temptation to take over because he knows that this would be counterproductive and the patients' development and independence would be unreasonably compromised.

Martin attempts to ensure that the weekly menu, drawn up by the patients, reflects at least one of the choices made by each individual. This activity calls for negotiating and, occasionally, arbitrating skills when trying to make sure that the menu reflects a balanced diet. The majority of the patients favour 'convenience' foods and appear to share Jack's view that 'The grub should be quick, hot and slide down easily!'. Martin and the team have to work at educating the patients so that this preference is balanced against the available budget and the need for a balanced diet.

Another factor that has to be attended to is the large amounts of tea, coffee and carbonated drinks consumed by some of the patients. In particular, Jack likes to drink at least 10 mugs of black coffee each day and insists on 'having the real stuff 'cos that decaffeinated stuff is rubbish'. This causes Jack to be restless and, at times, irritable. It also causes him to have palpitations and indigestion, resulting in him being frightened that he is having a heart attack. Whilst trying to educate Jack and help him to reduce his caffeine intake, Martin also has to reassure him when he becomes afraid and use strategies, such as relaxation therapy, exercise regimes and a reduction of environmental stimuli, to counteract Jack's restlessness, especially prior to bedtime.

Eliminating

This activity of daily living presents social as well as physical problems which requires Martin to use his communication skills as well as his observation skills. Communal living, as anyone from a large family will know, can give rise to difficulties, especially if there are a large number of people and a small number of toilet facilities. George finds it very frustrating when he cannot find a vacant toilet so he relieves himself in the garden – he justifies his actions by maintaining that 'it keeps the greenfly off the roses'. Martin not only has to try to deter Jack's behaviour but also has to respond to the neighbours' complaints. Once again, the skills of persuasion, tact and diplomacy come to the fore, which returns us to Jean's situation.

As outlined above, Jean is prone to constipation and this upsets her haemorrhoids. Apart from dealing sensitively with Jean in relation to ensuring that she has a regular bowel habit, has and uses medicaments for her haemorrhoids and is seen periodically by the general practitioner, Martin has to assess the effect that many of the other activities of living will have on Jean's condition and vice versa. For example:

- Eating and Drinking – high-fibre diet, adequate fluid intake
- Personal Cleansing and Dressing – ensuring that Jean does not wear restrictive clothing and regularly washes her anal area
- Mobilizing – making sure that Jean recognizes the importance of exercise and how it can adversely affect or enhance her condition.

Controlling body temperature

Body temperature is an important indicator of an individual's general state of health. Martin and his team are alert to this and monitor the patients for signs of any alteration from the normal body temperature, i.e. 37°C. Since a number of the patients are prescribed medication from the phenothiazine group, e.g., chlorpromazine, it is not unusual to find that some of them have a slightly lower temperature due to the effects of these drugs. This in itself is not of concern but it can mask the seriousness of an infection or inflammation. Therefore, any elevation in temperature must be compared to the individual's norm. For example, as indicated above, Harry is prone to chest infections. If he appears listless and complains of 'feeling off colour' and yet his temperature only appears to be slightly elevated, e.g. 37.4°C, this may not be seen as a cause for concern. However, it is known that Jack's usual temperature is only 36.2°C. Consequently, an increase is significant and would warrant the involvement of the general practitioner and possibly a course of antibiotics.

Another area, also related to the phenothiazines, which requires attention is that of photosensitivity. Therefore, patients who are taking these drugs, particularly chlorpromazine, need to be aware that they are at risk of serious sunburn. Once again, Martin and the team need to identify, educate and monitor those patients who are susceptible to this.

Mobilizing

Psychotropic drugs are also implicated in this activity in that one of the unwanted, and unpleasant, effects of some of these preparations is the production of Parkinsonims (musculoskeletal rigidity and tremor). Therefore, all patients taking these drugs need to be monitored and observed for signs of extra-pyramidal activity, e.g. mask-like expression, hand tremors, muscle spasm, shuffling gait. Should any of these occur, the medication regime will need to be reviewed, resulting in the reduction of the drug responsible or the addition/ increase of a preparation to counteract the unwanted effects, i.e. anticholinergics (rigidity and tremor controllers).

A general concern regarding mobilizing relates to the low level of physical activity displayed by some of the patients. Martin appreciates that enduring mental health problems often reduce motivation, volition and energy levels. These can be exacerbated by institutional living with the result that a number of patients appear content to do very little apart from sleep and generally lounge around. Encouragement is needed from the staff to ensure that these patients are involved in some appropriate exercise to maintain a reasonable level of physical fitness, e.g. walking, housework, gardening.

Working and playing

To maintain holistic health it is important to ensure that the activities and rewards gained from working and playing are balanced. As many of us know to our cost, this is easier said than done. At times one of these will dominate the other. For many of Martin's patients, 'playing' dominates their lives because the factors outlined in the above section coupled with the ever-present stigma of mental illness make it very difficult for the patients to find or retain paid employment. However, to enhance their self-esteem, increase self-worth and give them a sense of purpose and achievement, Martin assesses the patients for their suitability to attend a local sheltered workshop, makes referrals as appro-priate and ensures that support and encouragement are given to those who do attend.

Recreational activities in the house tend to revolve around the television and, although this could be seen loosely as a community activity, group activities are generally shunned by most patients. Appreciating the importance of living in harmony and the social, psychological benefits to be gained from retaining effec-tively with others, Martin endeavours to suggest and implement social activities both within and outside the house. Whilst a number of patients will engage in these activities when they are organized by the staff, few have the motivation, enthusiasm or confidence to be involved in the planning and running of events. This is well illustrated by Martin's suggestion that the patients might like to consider a day trip to France. Despite this being met by muted interest, it went ahead and generally appeared to be enjoyed, so much so that a few patients expressed interest in going again. However, when Martin tried to transfer the ownership for arranging the next trip to the patients, this was met with a blunt refusal despite staff help being offered. Martin is now trying to, slowly but surely, establish a position of 'working with' rather than 'doing for' the patients, so that independence and autonomy are promoted.

Expressing sexuality

Martin acknowledges that this activity of living warrants a great deal more attention than he and his team currently devote to it. Consistent with the observations made by Thomas (1989), sexuality is only addressed by the nurses when patients behave inappropriately, e.g. masturbating publicly, making unwanted sexual approaches to fellow patients. Because of this and the recognition that sexuality is notoriously difficult to define (Firn 1997), Martin has set up discussion sessions with the staff so that the nurses' role in relation to patients' sexual health can be explored. The main aims of this activity are to reduce staff embarrassment, educate staff in relation to practical advice for patients, e.g. safe sex, and develop a unit policy which will not only clarify the nurses' role but enable staff to consider the nurses' role but enable staff to consider sexuality in a broader, philosophical context, i.e. accepting that it is a multifaceted concept which involves biological, psychological, social, spiritual and cultural aspects. It is Martin's hope that when he and the team feel more comfortable and better equipped to deal effectively with sexuality, the patients can be supported more effectively and holistically.

Sleeping

Encountering problems with sleeping is very common in mental health settings and a number of the patients in Martin's unit experience some difficulty. These include inability to sleep, waking early, sleep disturbed by dreams/nightmares, somnambulism (sleepwalking), sleeping excessively and daytime sleeping adversely affecting the quality and duration of nighttime sleep.

Obviously, each patient's difficulties need to be assessed and responded to individually. However, some general factors need to be taken into consideration such as levels of activity, stress and stimulation, environmental factors such as heat, cold and noise, need for or reliance on hypnotic medication, eating and drinking habits, e.g. the ingestion of a heavy meal or beverage containing stimulants before retiring. Having identified which of these are affecting the patient and how, interventions, such as those outlined above for Jack, can be planned and implemented.

Dying

Rather like sexuality, this aspect tends to receive only limited attention and is only discussed when a specific issue arises. However, Martin recognizes that each patient has their own spiritual needs and, particularly as they increase in age, are likely to be more aware of their mortality. Efforts are made to allow each patient to practise their religious beliefs and if any of the patients appears to have concerns, fears or thoughts about dying they are encouraged to voice these and explore them with a member of the nursing team.

For example, Ted appeared to respond to the news of his sister's death in a quiet, matter-of-fact way but over the following two weeks he was observed on several occasions standing outside the local church staring at the stained glass window. When this was raised with him he at first dismissed this behaviour as being of no significance. However, Martin sensed that Ted was not only grieving for his sister but worrying about his own death. Through sensitive, supportive questioning, it was established that Ted was feeling afraid of when and how he might die. This was making him feel guilty because he felt he was putting his own 'selfish' needs above thoughts for his sister. Through a number of counselling sessions, Ted was helped to explore his situation and come to terms with both his loss and his fears for his own well-being.

By employing the main components of Roper *et al.*'s (1996) model, Martin's diverse responsibilities and range of skills have been illustrated. From this exploration of working with people suffering from enduring mental health problems it should be evident that, far from being a rather pedestrian, undemanding role, the work of the rehabilitation nurse demands high levels of observational skills, acute interaction and intervention skills and a great deal of motivation.

CARE OF THE ELDERLY

This section will offer a brief cast study as an introduction to caring for an older person, a description of an elderly care unit and the work of a mental health nurse working with clients with dementia.

It is important that effective care practices are crafted carefully and that love and warmth are valued and seen as being as real and important as physical needs. Any philosophy of care must integrate the training and caring needs of staff and reward good practice and caring regardless of a person's position in an organization (Morrissey and Coakley 1999).

Caring for older people has never held centre stage for health professionals (BMA 1986). However, it is important to recognize that nursing older people is challenging, stimulating and open to innovative ideas (White 1998). It also provides a profound platform to learn about caring and being cared for and an understanding of the meaning of people's lives as they were and as they unfold. At its most meaningful it allows nurses to enter the most private and vulnerable world of another person to explore and be with them through caring, living and loss. It is well recognized that the burden of care on mental health nurses and nursing assistants is heavy in such settings and burnout among caregivers is not uncommon (Almberg *et al.* 1997).

Care for people with dementia is on the increase and more than ever skilled mental health nurses are required at all levels (Morrissey and Coakley 1999). However, without the help of skilled nurses, caring nursing assistants and other health professionals, this will be impossible.

Dementia care is expensive, particularly for specialist care (Shah 1998), and unless radical changes occur, younger people with dementia will continue to receive services which are designed for older people (Keady and Matthews

1997). Of more concern is that a significant amount of care is administered by staff who have little if any formal training in working with older people (Bradshaw 1998), not to mention those with complex and distressing mental health problems, including depression (Bodnar *et al.* 1994).

Some individuals have very special nursing, medical and psychological needs requiring specialist input, including skilled mental health nurses. Clearly it is important that the development and promotion of good practice includes input from the elderly people whom we are meant to be serving (Rush *et al.* 1993).

More emphasis needs to be placed on psychological interventions with older people, including the use of appropriate neuropsychological tests (Lichtenberg 1998). There is also a need to at least identify the needs of people from different ethnic and cultural backgrounds (Tilki 1994).

The spiritual needs of all individuals need careful and serious consideration given the need for people to understand their lives and try to come to terms with profound issues like change, illness, death, bereavement and loneliness. This need is echoed by recent research which stresses the need for nurses to recognize this and other issues. In many elderly units individuals may come from different cultures and hold different religious or spiritual beliefs, for example muslim, jewish or another faith. Given the diversity of care required and the increasing provision of care by private community homes it is important to illustrate some common themes relating to elderly care with particular reference to dementia care. An elderly unit will be briefly outlined and the work of one staff nurse will be discussed in the light of current care practices.

CASE STUDY 9.1

Maria remembered her mother Catherine as she used to be: a gentle woman always there to support her children and a very dear friend. Maria remembered growing up with her brothers and sisters. More importantly, Maria was aware of the moments that had marked their very special mother–daughter relationship.

Now at 76 Catherine was clearly a very different person who experienced gradual, significant, psychological changes. The first was her failing ability to do the shopping but then there came hostility which was totally out of character. Later Catherine became more hostile to Maria who was now aware that something was not quite right with her mother. However, it was only after a visit to her GP that Alzheimer's disease was first mentioned and months later before it was confirmed. The following two years marked a significant deterioration in her memory to such an extent that she forgot where she was and sometimes would call Maria to attend to her but would then be in a muddle. At times Catherine had lost all the qualities that Maria knew as her mother which made caring all the more difficult.

Four years after her mother's death, Maria still feels things could have been better dealt with and still the grief lies just below the surface. What was very difficult was finding respite care as Maria insisted that her mother be cared for at home. Eventually Maria accepted the use of Denton House.

Denton House

Denton House, a 40-bed unit, was commissioned as a purpose-built home for the elderly with mental health problems mainly associated with Alzheimer's disease. These clients would need long-term medical and nursing care. Strict admission criteria had been agreed with the health authority so that people who needed to be admitted were formally assessed and matched the criteria before admission was agreed. Prior to the building of this home older people with mental health problems from a set geographical area were cared for on two psychiatric wards in the local hospital.

The home was opened in 1994 and needed to be established with staff, including a housekeeper team and catering staff.

Trained staff

The majority were recruited from the local psychiatric hospital, establishing a core staff which had formal training in mental health and experience in care of the elderly with mental health problems. Some were general nurses with an interest in working with elderly people.

Untrained staff

A few staff came from elderly wards within the trust with little mental health background or experience in dealing with older people with mental health problems. Other care staff came from the private sector, namely nursing homes, and there were some with little or no experience of care work.

A staff nurse at Denton House

What is immediately striking about Denton House is that staff don't wear uniform and that it is modern and purpose built. There are two long corridors and each floor has separate staff and residents. Other basic features are that you need a number to unlock the front door and some door locks have been put in to prevent people wandering off the unit.

Michael Lawrence is 26 years old and has been working as a staff nurse at Denton House for two years. Michael primarily works with clients with dementia. The next few paragraphs will outline some of the work involved in day-to-day care with an insight into some of the nursing issues.

> *Sometimes I wonder whether I will get through another day as the work is so physically and emotionally draining. I can really identify with the despair and loneliness carers must feel. You really have to want to do this work yet I know however bad I am feeling that my skills as a mental health nurse make a difference in the lives of those I care for. (Michael)*

The main aspect of Michael's work is working with carers, nurses, doctors and other health professionals. It is useful to draw on the above case study to illustrate how care is organized. Michael is involved in home assessments, usually with another member of the team, sometimes a doctor. The team assesses the person's ability to selfcare and the carer, in this case Maria's, ability and motivation to supplement it. It was evident that Maria enjoyed and felt it a duty to care for her mother, especially in relation to personal care.

> *I don't see it as a job as I love my mother and she has given so much to me, and yes, it is terribly sad to leave her to the mercy of others who don't know her as she was not so very long ago.*
>
> *Sometimes I have confided to Michael the enormous strain I am under but really I don't feel I could sleep if I did anything else. I realize that one day she may need to stay in Denton House but until then I will struggle on. (Maria)*

Michael delivers nursing care to 40 residents, a small proportion of whom are there for respite care but the majority for round-the-clock care. Clearly, when in this role Michael has to organize staff and ensure that care plans are appropriate. Follow-up includes helping carers deal with crisis points including referrals and organizing home visits. At Denton House staff support is provided in the form of an open group with a facilitator from outside. Other facilities include a carers' group and family days to inform and support families caring for an elderly relative. However, the demands of caring take their toll on all staff.

> *I sometimes feel everyone wants a bit of me and it is hard to get the balance right. We need to take care of ourselves better. I would not offer advice to newly qualified staff except to recognize that your partner, family and friends also need to be cared for and loved. Mainstream nurse training or medical training can never prepare you totally for the experience of caring for the older person particularly those with dementia. (Michael)*

Some issues in care

Catherine's care
Monitoring:

- cognitive skills and abilities
- affect or mood state
- behaviour
- her physical well-being.

Promote:

- independence
- activity, rest and sleep
- sufficient nutritional intake
- respect and dignity
- social contact with significant others
- interests or hobbies or contact with pets
- psychological and spiritual well-being
- support from others including staff
- friendship and family involvement in care

- communication with self and others
- personal care
- partnerships in care
- support for family and children.

Maria's care

- Assess informational needs *re* Alzheimer's disease.
- Assess understanding of care demand and progress of Alzheimer's disease and commitment and ability to care.
- Identify deficits or gaps in care. Identify support available to Maria. Assess family level of support with clear picture of roles and resources, particularly emotional issues around grief and bereavement. Key worker to help Maria to deal with the changes taking place in her mother.
- Help Maria to identify pace of care including her need for emotional and psychological support.

Staff

- Communication between staff to be involved.
- Arranging and coordinating the compiling of records with review dates including staff team and key worker.
- Planning respite care and identifying facilities in advance.

Challenges faced by staff nurses in dementia care are mainly in relation to the short-term and long-term quality of care for people with or affected by dementia.

Recent discussion has surrounded the clinical challenges faced by nurses in dementia care and also those faced by carers and nurses (Kitwood 1997, Morrissey and Coakley 1999). The main themes in the literature are lack of appropriately trained nurses to provide nursing care and the general lack of training in dealing with older people and specifically those with dementia (Bradshaw 1998). Some of the main concerns for nursing include lack of staff, lack of basic privacy and care for residents. There are some examples of good practice in elderly care and dementia care yet providing a stable workforce in this environment is difficult.

Novel ways to provide social support and human contact are family days and carers-support groups. Some homes have a cat or dog (Dembicki and Anderson 1996) and visits from children have positive therapeutic consequences for elderly people. Such visits can also help children come to terms with old age and loss (Magnuson 1999, Morrissey 1999). The use of music can also help staff build closer relationships with residents and each other (Suzuki 1998). Some managers have followed a more integrated model or philosophy of nursing care which reflects both staff and resident needs.

In dementia care, there is a need to protect the person's safety, e.g. from self-harm or injury, while promoting contact with others who have a good relationship with that person. It is all too easy to stop communicating with a person because they are not able to respond coherently or verbally.

The lead often comes from the family carer but also from the bond between staff in a particular home who can be a role model to all of us. It is important to recognize the importance of humour and other human qualities in improving the lives of carers and clients. Respect is a quality which should not be seen as automatic but should be offered in a thoughtful and considered way. Therapies need to be provided by occupational therapists and clinical psychologists which can free time for staff to provide dignified nursing care and therapy.

Care of older people can be innovative and rewarding yet investment in people must include all those who work in this area, including the support of nursing assistants. Health promotion in elderly care has been reviewed (Young 1998) yet the health of staff must also be addressed: physical, psychological, emotional and spiritual. Health care in the future needs to tackle the burden of care faced by families (Feely 1997) and help them to plan ahead.

CONCLUSION

As stated at the beginning of this chapter, four main areas of nursing care have been covered with a view to identifying the main skills used by nurses in each. It should have become apparent that there is no one way to care – each nurse will bring to the client their own expertise and an individual understanding of the needs of the client

Nowhere is this more true than in the community, where nurses, often working alone or on a one-to-one basis with the client, will quickly prioritize care. Care is undertaken with the help of the client, carers and other members of the team and referrals to others should be made when appropriate but the community mental health nurse is very often the channel through which the others are directed.

REFERENCES

Almberg, B., Graftstrom, M. and Winblad, B. (1997) Caring for a demented elderly person: burden and burnout among caregiving relatives. *Journal of Advanced Nursing* 25(1): 109–116.

Ash, J. (1997) Psychological assessment and measurement. In: Thomas, B., Hardy, S. and Cutting, P. (eds) *Stuart and Sundeen's Mental Health Nursing: Principles and Practice*. Mosby, London.

Barker, P. (1997) *Assessment in Psychiatric and Mental Health Nursing*. Stanley Thornes, Cheltenham.

Bodnar, J.C., Kiecolt, G. and Janice, K. (1994) Caregiver depression after bereavement: chronic stress isn't over when it's over. *Psychology and Aging* 9(3): 372–380.

Boyd, M. and Nihart, M. (1998) *Psychiatric Nursing: contemporary practice*. Lippincott, Philadelphia.

Bradshaw, A. (1998) Charting some challenges in the art and science of nursing. *Lancet* 351(9100): 438–440.

British Medical Association (1986) *All Our Tomorrows: growing old in Britain*. BMA. London.

Cormack, D. (1983) *The Research Process in Nursing*. Blackwell Science, Oxford.

Cutting, P. (1997) Concepts, models and theories in psychiatric and mental health nursing. In: Thomas, B., Hardy, S. and Cutting, P. (eds) *Mental Health Nursing*. Mosby, London.

Dembicki, D. and Anderson, J. (1996) Pet ownership may be a factor in improved health of the elderly. *Journal of Nutrition for the Elderly*. 15(3): 15–31.

DoH (1994) *Working in Partnership*. HMSO, London.

Falloon, I. (1988) *Handbook of Behavioral Family Therapy*. Guilford Press, New York.

Feely, J. (1997) Alzheimer's disease. *Health Which?* 6: 172–173.

Firn, S. (1997) Key issues in sexual health. In: Thomas, B., Hardy, S. and Cutting, P. (eds) *Stuart and Sundeen's Mental Health Nursing: Principles and Practice*. Mosby, London.

Forster, S. (ed.) (1997) *The A–Z of Community Mental Health Practice*. Stanley Thornes, Cheltenham.

Gamble, C. (1993) Working with schizophrenic patients and their families. *British Journal of Nursing* 2(17): 856–859.

Hargie, O. (ed.) (1997) *The Handbook of Communication Skills*. Routledge, London.

Heron, J. (1997) *Dimensions of Facilitator Style*. Human Potential Resource Group, University of Surrey.

Jackman, C. (1991) The experience and psychological impact of early miscarriage. *Irish Journal of Psychology* 12(2): 108–120.

Janosik, E. (1996) *Mental Health and Psychiatric Nursing*. Little, Brown, Boston.

Keable, D. (1989) *The Management of Anxiety: a manual for therapists*. Churchill Livingstone, Edinburgh.

Keady, J. and Matthews, L. (1997) Younger people with dementia. *Elderly Care* 9(4): 19–23.

Kitwood, T. (1997) *Dementia Reconsidered*. Open University Press, Buckinghamshire.

Libermann, R. (1992) *Handbook of Psychiatric Rehabilitation*. Macmillan, Basingstoke.

Lichtenberg, P. (1998) Cost-effective geriatric neuropsychology. In: Hartman-Stein, P.E. *et al.* (eds) *Innovative Behavioral Healthcare for Older Adults: a guidebook for changing times*. Jossey-Bass, San Francisco, pp. 79–102.

Magnuson, S. (1999) Strategies to help students whose grandparents have Alzheimer's disease. *Professional School Counseling* 2(4): 327–333.

Maslow, A. (1962) *Towards a Psychology of Being*. Van Nostrand, Princeton.

Morrissey, M.V. (1999) Love, loss and disappearing lives. In: Morrissey, M.V. and Coakley, A.L. (1999) *Alzheimer's Disease: beyond the medical model*. Quay Books, Mark Allen Publishers, Salisbury, Wiltshire.

Morrissey, M.V. and Coakley, A.L. (1999) *Alzheimer's Disease: beyond the medical model*. Quay Books, Mark Allen Publishers, Salisbury, Wiltshire.

Nelson-Jones, R. (1993) *Practical Counselling and Helping Skills*. Cassell, London.

NHSE (1996) *Guidance on Supervised Discharge (Aftercare under Supervision) and Related Provisions*. NHSE, London.

Peplau, H. (1952) *Interpersonal Relations in Nursing*. Putman, New York.

Roper, N., Logan, W. and Tierney, A. (1996) *The Elements of Nursing*. Churchill Livingstone, Edinburgh.

Rush, B., Molloy, D. and Harrison, C. (1993) The erosion of autonomy in long-term care. *Canadian Medical Association Journal* 149(6): 845–846.

Segal, L. (1991) *Slow Motion*. Virago, London.

Shah, A. (1998) Dementia and dementia care. *International Journal of Geriatric Psychiatry* 13(1): 67.

Sherr, L. (1995) *The Psychology of Pregnancy and Childbirth*. Blackwell Science, Oxford.

Stewart, A. (1994) *At a Loss. Bereavement Care When a Baby Dies*. Baillière Tindall, London.

Suzuki, A.I. (1998) The effects of music therapy on mood and congruent memory of elderly adults with depressive symptoms. *Music Therapy Perspectives* 16(2): 75–80.

Thomas, B. (1989) Asexual patients. *Nursing Times* 85(33): 49–51.

Tilki, M. (1994) Ethnic Irish older people. *British Journal of Nursing* 3(17): 909–913.

Towell, D. (1975) *Innovations in Patient Care*. Croom Helm, London.

Winefield, H. and Harvey, R. (1994) Determinants of psychological distress in relatives of people with chronic schizophrenia. *Schizophrenia Bulletin* 19(3): 619–625.

Wykes, T. (1993) *Violence and Health Care Professionals*. Chapman and Hall, London.

White, C. (1998) Age no bar to a caring career ... caring for elderly people. *Nursing Times* 94(29): 69–72.

Young, K. (1998) Health and health promotion in the elderly. *Journal of Clinical Nursing* 5(4): 241–248.

INDEX